SUPPORT FROM SCIENTISTS, INDUSTRY AND THE CULTURING COALITION

From the Scientific Community

"This amazing book has restored my excitement for truly natural whole food supplements with its research and dispelled my skepticism with its excellent review of medical literature."

> —Jesse Hanley, M.D., Author of *Tired of Being Tired* (Putnam, 2001), medical educator and best-selling author after twenty years of private practice in Malibu, CA.

"Wow, I've never read a more in-depth, well researched and detailed explanation of the physiology of nutrients. I learned a lot! Anyone considering taking a supplement should read this first."

> —Christine Horner, M.D., F.A.C.S., host and medical editor of nationally syndicated news segment "Natural Health Insights." Author of the upcoming book *A Plastic Surgeon's Secrets: How to Slow the Aging Process, Enhance Your Beauty and Stay Healthy Naturally.*

"*Life Bridge* is a long overdue introduction to the important role the culturing process has played, and continues to play, in human health and nutrition. The book illustrates that nutrition is more than the sum of its separate parts, and that through the process of culturing, a synergy of health promoting compounds is created. The recent trend in nutrition has been to take a linear "more is better" approach by concentrating specific vitamins or minerals in pharmacological quantities. This book demonstrates some of the fallacies in this unbalanced approach to nutrition, and suggests a new paradigm of nutrition where "less is more" and health is not a function of quantity but of quality."

> —Gregory Kelly, N.D., Instructor of Clinical Nutrition, University of Bridgeport, College of Naturopathic Medicine, Associate Editor of Alternative Medicine Review

"*Life Bridge* presents powerful medical evidence illustrating the safety and efficacy of probiotic nutrients. This is an excellent nutritional guide for doctors and patients alike."

> —Lyn Yaffe, M.D., Commander, Navy Medical Corps, Retired. Previously, Director, Research and Development, Naval Medical Research and Development Command, United States Navy

"I have been in the fermentation business for over twenty five years. After reading this book, I have a greater appreciation for the profound wisdom of our ancestors who have practiced this art and made it a part of their daily life. The science of probiotics and the wisdom of using more bioavailable forms of vitamins and minerals has been meticulously explained in simple words. You have managed to explain a very complicated subject so beautifully. It was a treat for me to read this book!"

> —Dr. N. Suresh, PhD, Biochemistry, Madurai University, India, Post-doctoral research, Molecular Biology and Microbiology, Tufts University Medical School and Brandeis University, pharmaceutical and fermentation scientist

"A persuasive argument for probiotic whole-food supplements."

> —Dr. David C.Radford, DC, DAAPM, Associate Staff, Lutheran Hospital Cleveland Clinic, Spine Center

"A compelling scientific case for the use of probiotic whole-food nutrition for the maintenance of health."
—Radha Maheshwari, PhD, Professor of Pathology at a leading
US medical school and research institution

"I have had great success incorporating probiotic whole-food nutrients into my medical practice, and I'm pleased to recommend *"Life Bridge"* to my professional colleagues. It is a concise yet thorough treatment of the medical value of probiotic nutrients, and it may well breathe new life into the way the medical community approaches nutritional supplementation."
—Philip M. Lichtenfeld, M.D., FAAFP, Medical Director,
Beverly Hills Doctors Medical Associates, Inc.

"*The Life Bridge* makes it crystal clear that whole foods or probiotic whole foods are the best possible source for nutrients for our bodies."
—Robert Blaesing, R.Ph.

"The scientific information as related to food and nutrients was wonderful information to educate my patients about changing their eating habits to live healthier and longer lives."
—Hal Stein, D.C., FIAMA

"As a retired scientist who spent a better part of my life in food research and development, I can only applaud and support the work of Dr. Sarnat, Schulick and Newmark. This is probably one of the most important pieces of work for the people of the 21st century. With optimal nutrition on the decline, food sources challenged by a polluted environment and disease rampant, it is my hope that every person today has the fortune of reading and embracing the concepts of *The Life Bridge*."
—Dr. Pio Angelini, Analytical Chemist in Food Science
Laboratory of Pioneering Research, Natick Army Research and
Development Command, Over 40 years of service to science

From our Friends in the Culturing Coalition

"As the science of health develops, we are becoming increasingly aware that vast communities of microorganisms are enlisted to aid homeostasis. Fermented foods are the vanguard of good nutrition. What this book accomplishes so superbly is the revealing that microbial allies potentate our health and host defenses."
—Paul Stamets, mycologist, author of *Growing Gourmet & Medicinal Mushrooms*, founder of Fungi Perfecti, and research associate with the
Program for Integrative Medicine at the University of Arizona

"This is a well written book that makes the scientific case for what we knew anecdotally—that cultured foods enhance our health and happiness."
—Steve Ford, Pres., Brown Cow Farm, www.browncowfarm.com

"The miracle of natural fermentation transforms the bitter cacao seed into the stuff that dreams are made of: fine chocolate. Through fermentation, the flavors, aromas, and polyphenols of cacao are brought to life, and *Life Bridge* explains how fermentation works the same magic for all probiotic nutrients. I highly recommend *Life Bridge* for health-conscious consumers (together with some Moonstruck Chocolate, of course)."
—Anthony Roth, President and CEO, Moonstruck Chocolate

"This book confirms what humankind has known intuitively for several millennia: Properly brewed beer is good for you. The only difference is that the authors are able to explain why this is the case."
—Tom Schlafly, a recovering lawyer who found true fulfillment when he opened the first microbrewery in St. Louis in 1991, The Saint Louis Brewery and Tap Room

"Scientists now believe that humanity's most ancient cultivated plants are not grains and vegetables but rather microscopic organisms— molds, yeast, and bacteria—that cause foods to ferment. Modern research is just beginning to realize the incredible healing power of fermented foods. *The Life Bridge*, by Richard L. Sarnat, M.D., Paul Schulick, and Thomas M. Newmark, is a major contribution to the our understanding of the importance of the miracle of fermentation."
—John Belleme, American Miso Company.

"I would never have thought of the existence of *The Life Bridge* without this enlightening text but now somehow it all seems to make perfect sense! How wonderful that there are organisms around willing and able to build these bioavailability bridges for us. As a vegan it's very reassuring to know that my daily tempeh is providing me with the valuable and elusive vitamin B-12 I need."
—Polly Syred, Phytofoods/Tempeh Kits, Microscopix Publications

"A lovely book explaining the unique health benefits of probiotic whole food. Well worth reading while sipping a cup of tea."
—Ron Rubin, The Minister of Tea, The Republic of Tea
He is also the author, with Stuart Avery Gold, of *Success@Life* (2001, NewmarketPress)

"Congratulations to the authors. What a remarkable compilation of information on cultured foods. *The Life Bridge* allows people interested in cultured foods to have access to a multi-faceted overview that is responsibly and impressively researched.
As founder of Rejuvenative Foods (we've been offering Raw Cultured Vegetables in the refrigerated sections of natural food stores since 1980); I appreciate reading about the benefits of raw cultured vegetables and yogurt stated in *The Life Bridge* and I am very pleased about the clarification that Raw Cultured Vegetables are a delicious beneficial source of *lactobacillus* and enzymes; for all people including those wishing an alternative to yogurt."
—Evan Richards, founder Rejuvenative Foods
www. rejuvenative.com; email: mail@rejuvenative.com

"Since reading *The Life Bridge*, my morning cup of coffee has never tasted healthier. This well-written book provides the reader with a fascinating scientific perspective on the foods and beverages we consume everyday, and provides more than its share of surprises along the way."
—Rick Peyser, Green Mountain Coffee Roasters
www.GreenMountainCoffee.com

"We all know that wine brings joy, and now the authors of *Life Bridge* explain why wine, one of the great cultured foods, brings health. When science meets pleasure, it's time to celebrate. To *Life Bridge*, I say "cheers!""
—Doug Margerum, Wine Cask, Santa Barbara, California

From our Friends in the Natural Products Industry

"In *Life Bridge* the authors have presented a lyrical and scientifically sound position on the value of cultured foods and cultured vitamins and minerals. With thorough research information and a thorough understanding of human nutritional history, they have created their own bridge between traditional wisdom and modern scientific method. The result is sure to enlighten and educate several generations-from the "Baby Boomers" through "Generation X" and beyond."
> —Kathy Svoboda, National Natural Living Sales
> and Training Manager Wild Oats Market, Inc.

"For centuries it has been well known that almost all the advanced and primitive societies have used cultured foods products. Several groups that use cultured products have some of the longer life expectancies. Now recent research proves that culturing supplements with foods makes the nutrients more bio-available. I think this is exciting new information to the benefit of the health food customer."
> —Joseph M. Bassett, President, Bassett Health Foods, Inc., Toledo, Ohio,
> and Past President, National Nutritional Foods Association (NNFA)

"We at Rainbow Blossom are strong proponents of cultured foods, such as miso, tempeh, yogurt, and probiotic whole-food vitamins and minerals. Culturing optimizes nutrients for maximum health benefit, and this wonderful new book explains in clear terms why this is so. I applaud this important contribution to the science of nutrition."
> —Rob Auerbach, owner of The Rainbow Blossom Stores based in
> Louisville, KY, *Whole Foods Magazine* Retailer of the Year

"This book makes a convincing case for the founding principle of the natural products industry: the best nourishment comes from traditionally prepared whole foods. We now understand that culturing vitamins and minerals takes them across the "Life Bridge," and makes them more bioavailable and effective. *Life Bridge* is a must read for all health-conscious consumers."
> —Phil Nabors, owner of The Mustard Seed Stores based in
> Cleveland, OH, *Whole Foods Magazine* Retailer of the Year

"An important and innovative book that assists consumers in understanding the origins of and relationships between food and nutritional supplementation. The authors provide a "bridge" which allows the reader to better appreciate the reality and significant benefits that have been gained from current nutritional knowledge while at the same time, allowing them to cross into the future and recognize the need to develop additional health strategies, alternatives and nutritional products for the future."
> —R. Mark Stowe, Licensed Nutritionist, owner of
> Nutrition Cottage, Delray Beach, Florida.

"*Life Bridge . . . The Way to Longevity with Probiotic Nutrients*, provides a thoughtful and elegant approach to staying healthy naturally. Those of us who are passionate about participating in this great search for natural (and safer) healing methods would do well to consider honestly the words of the authors who state: 'The answer lies somewhere within the mystery of living whole food'. This book provides compelling details on why we should not only eat the best foods possible but also why we should supplement our diets with probiotic nutrients. The authors write in a style that is accessible to the scientific researcher and general public alike. The evidence is quite convincing in favor of what they call 'the decision to have the living nutrients work with us.' Yes!!"
> —Michael Kanter, Cambridge Naturals, Cambridge, MA

"A great primer on the health benefits of cultured foods and vitamins and a nice departure from USP isolated vitamins to whole food nutrients. A great book."

—John Nelson, Vitamin Manager, Mother's Market & Kitchen

"What a wisdom filled and timely book! As a professional member of the American Herbalists Guild specializing in Ayurveda and with 28 years of running Smile Herb Shop, a retail herb store, I have had access to just about all the products and theories available today. *The Life Bridge* continues the excellent contribution Paul Schulick and Tom Newmark make to the healing of our culture. Time will uphold deeper wisdom in healing and "Life Bridge" will prove to be a classic text speeding our crossing to such depth."

—Tom Wolf, owner, Smileherb.com, member American Herbalists Guild

"What a cutting edge, innovative work! Scientific integrity and common sense, what a noval idea! Well thought, well researched, well written, WELL DONE! *The Life Bridge* is a "must read" for any practitioner."

—Jack Cluney, Ph.D., President HealthSource, Inc.,
Nutritional Wellness Center

"*The Life Bridge* so beautifully supports information we have been offering people about nutrition in general and specifically whole foods for years in all of our stores. The depth of the information involved now gives us a chance to be much more detailed with people than we've ever been before about the reality and value of whole food nutrition. The marriage between this information, how it's been presented and our all organic food services is something I hadn't expected to see for quite sometime."

—Seth Alan Siegel, owner & CEO Health Emporium Market,
Grilles, and Clinics, Corona Del Mar, CA

"Eloquently and passionately written, *The Life Bridge* is the science behind the importance of cultured foods. If we wish to live long, healthy, and vibrant lives, the wisdom of our ancestors needs to penetrate deeply into our diets of today. This book spoke to my heart, I now look at foods and nutritional supplements with new awareness. I loved this book, and need to read it again and probably again."

—Linda Howes, CN, 14 Carrots, New London, NH

From Our Friends in the Media

"*The Life Bridge* is thick and sweet with insight, profoundly compelling arguments, and enjoyable, well reasoned, and well-researched narrative. The authors use the bright spotlight of a finely honed pen to show you the wisdom of ancient foods. After reading halfway through, I immediately went to the cupboard and took some organic miso. Later, I had some brewers yeast in juice. Get the picture? *The Life Bridge* has helped me see something important and new."

—Paul Schaefer, Wisdom Television Network

"Once again Tom, Paul and Rick have put out an important work that demystifies the natural products industry confusion. *Life Bridge* sets the record straight, going back through history to prove it isn't nice to fool Mother Nature. Humans need food, whole food. This is the ABC's of cultured food. This book tells the truth, the whole truth."

—Frankie Boyer, host of *The Business of Being Healthy* radio show

Here with a Loaf of Bread beneath the Bough,
A Flask of Wine, a Book of Verse—and Thou
Beside me singing in the Wilderness—
And Wilderness is Paradise enow.
—*Rubaiyat of Omar Khayyam*

The Life Bridge

The Way to Longevity
With Probiotic Nutrients

By
Richard L. Sarnat, M.D.
Paul Schulick, and
Thomas M. Newmark

Notice

The Life Bridge: The Way to Longevity with Probiotic Nutrients is for informational purposes only, and is not a guide for the treatment of any individual's disease or medical condition. The authors hope that the book will provide valuable information about the latest developments in nutritional science and holistic healthcare, and will stimulate consideration of medical options. Because every person is different, however, a qualified physician must diagnose conditions and recommend or supervise the use of healing foods for the treatment of any health problems. Herbs, other natural remedies, and cultured foods are not substitutes for professional medical care. You should consult a qualified health care practitioner familiar with your medical condition and history before using any of the cultured foods or recommendations in this book. You should seek the best medical guidance to make your decisions informed and most effective in promoting health. At various points in the book, portions of quoted text have been put in boldface.

The Life Bridge

The Way to Longevity
With Probiotic Nutrients

By
Richard L. Sarnat, M.D.
Paul Schulick, and
Thomas M. Newmark

Herbal Free Press
Brattleboro, VT

OTHER BOOKS BY THE AUTHORS

Ginger: Common Spice and Wonder Drug
by **Paul Schulick**

Beyond Aspirin: Nature's Answer to Arthritis
Cancer and Alzheimer's Disease
by **Thomas Newmark and Paul Schulick**

Physician Heal Thyself: What Every Practitioner
Should Know About Alternative Medicine
by **Richard Sarnat, M.D.**

ACKNOWLEDGEMENTS

The creation of this book benefited from the support and assistance of a number of enthusiastic fans of probiotic nutrients. Herb Lewis and Nancy Angelini, nationally prominent health educators and leaders of the complementary medical movement, generously contributed their knowledge about the value of probiotic nutrition, and much of the book was directly inspired by their suggestions. Jen Toomey helped enormously in the creation of the graphs and tables for the book, and Shukyo Lin Pfleger, Jewel Hernandez, and Kathie Robinson endured our endless edits as they laid out the book and readied it for publication. Shukyo also designed the cover and is responsible for what we think is a lovely layout and look. Connie Tumavicus kindly assisted in the editing and proofing of the book, and Kelli Rooney offered valuable guidance in the organization of materials, especially the design of the reference section. We thank Terry Newmark for the illustration introducing each chapter. Most of all, we thank the unnamed and unknown custodians of probiotic cultures throughout the ages, who tenderly guarded our *Life Bridge* allies and preserved them for the benefit of all humankind.

DEDICATION

The authors dedicate this book to their
fathers—loving men, devoted to science,
scholarship, plants, and family.
Thank you Leonard, Raymond, and Melvin.
The heroes are alive so long as the
poets still sing of them.

TABLE OF CONTENTS

"Fermentation is the oldest known form of food biotechnology; records of barley conversion to beer date back more than 5000 years.... The traditional fermentation of food serves several functions, [including] enrichment of food substrates biologically with protein, essential amino acids, essential fatty acids, and vitamins...."
—Food and Agricultural Organization of the United Nations, Rome 1999

"There are numerous studies showing fermentation of food with lactobacilli increase the quantity, availability, digestibility, and assimilability of nutrients."
—*Lactic Acid Bacteria and Human Health,* Tufts University School of Medicine

probiotic (pro-bi-ot′ik). Relating to probiosis. An association of two organisms that enhances the life process of both.
—Stedman Medical Dictionary, 25th Edition

PROBIOTIC FACTS
"...The number of microbial cells in the body is 10-20 times larger (10^{14}) than the total number of eukaryotic cells in the whole body (10^{13})....

...An indication of the complexity of the flora and its numerous metabolic functions is the observation that the flora of an individual contains approximately 300,000 genes, compared with approximately 65,000 in the rest of the body...."

—*Curr Opin Clin Nutr Metab Care* 2001;4(6):571-9. Pre-, pro- and synbiotics. Bengmark S. Department of Hepatology and Surgery, University College of London, Liver Institute. PubMed UI: 11706296

INTRODUCTION

The three of us who are writing this have been friends for over thirty years. In our respective careers, we are an MD and surgeon, herbal scientists, organic farmers, founder of an extensive integrative medical network, owners of a nutritional company, and, perhaps most importantly, we are all products of the 1950s. "Baby Boomers." Many of you reading this share that identity, or have parents of that generation. We were bottle fed because it was thought to be more civilized and nourishing than nursing from our mothers' breasts. We were routinely dosed with antibiotics because modern science deemed that better than letting our young bodies build their own immune defenses. Surgeons routinely removed our tonsils, for after all, those organs weren't really necessary. We were dressed in polyesters and synthetics because they could keep their crease, even in hot weather! We learned in amazement that astronauts could eat and drink powdered synthetic nutrients in space, and we yearned to be just like them. We wore spacesuits at Halloween, we watched the Jetsons, we named a baseball team the "Astros," and we replaced messy natural grass with "Astroturf." Is it any wonder that we were told, and we believed, that Tang® was better for us than orange juice and that the fortified refined flour of Wonder Bread® would make our bodies stronger and healthier

—in twelve ways!—than the grains of our ancestors? Those were the days when Science trumped Nature, and pharmaceutical companies trumped kitchens. Father may have known best, but Mother Nature was antiquated compared to gleaming laboratories. White powder replaced green healing, and the Age of Mega-Potency Vitamins was upon us. So began a paradigm of nutrition that led to the ultimate vanity: *Nutrients purified from the earth or isolated from whole food were better than the whole food itself.*

We reject that paradigm. It is our firm medical and scientific judgment, based on thousands of years of human nutritional experience and countless scientific confirmations, that probiotic whole food, as traditionally consumed, is the best form of nourishment for humankind. That is not to say that we reject nutritional supplementation, for we do not. Our farms and grocery stores are in large part failing to deliver the living nutrients so needed in our polluted and stressful times, so we acknowledge that mineral and vitamin supplementation is an important health strategy. We are convinced, however, that such supplementation should strive to deliver nutrients in a probiotic whole-food form, much as food biotechnology has wisely and safely employed for over 5000 years. As the *United Nations Rome Report* of 1999 correctly assessed, the culturing of whole food leads to the "enrichment of nutritive content by microbial synthesis of essential vitamins and improving digestibility of protein and carbohydrates." And the experience of civilizations for thousands of years confirms that probiotic nutrients are an invaluable ally for humankind. This book will examine the substantial tradition and science supporting the use of probiotic whole food nutrients, and it will conclude with a call to return to the timeless wisdom of probiotic foods. We will in *Chapter Three*, take a light dip into the biochemistry of probiotic foods, and *Chapters Four* and *Five* will explore individual nutrients and contrast the varying forms of available supplementation. But before we get practical and physical, we will begin this book with the "metaphysics," the very origins, of food.

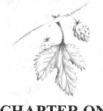

CHAPTER ONE

The Miracle of Life

It is in and by means of the cell that the molecular world
'appears in person' (if I may so express myself), touch-
ing, passing into, and disappearing into the higher con-
structions of life.
　—Father Teilhard de Chardin,
　　The Phenomenon of Man

When it happened, perhaps only God or the mystics
know. But life emerged out of inorganic matter, and from
that the "Phenomenon of Man" occurred. We appreciate
the miracle of life, but we have never been able to dupli-
cate it in a laboratory. Those first, microscopic life forms
may stand at the shimmering edge of pure inorganic
matter, but they are more different from chemicals than
they are from humans. They, like we, are alive.

If you gave every Nobel laureate unlimited resources
and an eternity, does anyone think that our finest minds
could create life out of inorganic matter? Of course not—
it is simply beyond human understanding. And in the
evolutionary chain decreed by whatever force or forces
that set life in motion, one thing is clear: humans eat food.
We have never eaten purified, isolated, or synthesized
minerals or naked molecules. Instead, we have drawn

nourishment from either plants or other animals, and that living food is more than the sum of its inorganic parts. It is infused with the organizing brilliance of life itself.

Standing at the edge of matter and forming the first link in the chain of life are simple life forms as Brewer's yeast (*Saccharomyces cerevisiae*) and various beneficial bacteria such as *Lactobacillus acidophilus*, *L. bifidus*, and *L. rhamnosus*. By their incorporation and transformation of inorganic matter, they create nourishment that has sustained human life for millennia. And that process is most commonly called "culturing."

We will be considering individual minerals and vitamins in *Chapters Four* and *Five* and exploring how their probiotic form is, for humans, the superior form of nourishment. Before that, however, we would like to spend a few moments in tribute to the process of culturing itself. It is ancient, certainly more ancient than human life. Paleontologists have determined that our Paleolithic ancestors had a million times more living *Lactobacillus plantarum* in their digestive systems than do we, a function perhaps of our eating processed and lifeless foods or inert chemicals. More fundamentally, our very digestive systems are constructed on the process of culturing, for our "symbiotic" relationship with probiotics ensures that all of our foods are ultimately "cultured" within our digestive system. In fact, we know that many food nutrients simply are unavailable to humans unless our probiotic allies are properly functioning. Such is the interplay in the chain of life.

How do these simple life forms interact with inorganic matter? We have vague notions, but not hard answers. We know for example that Brewer's yeast has at least seven different protein systems for bringing elemental iron into its cells. In a 1999 special article in *Nutrition Reviews* entitled "Iron Transport Across Biologic Membranes," research scientists from Children's Hospital in Boston report that:

> Organisms have developed a variety of strategies for solubilizing iron and transporting it into cells. Because iron is toxic in excess, transport is meticulously regulated and chelating compounds are produced to detoxify both extracellular and intracellular iron.... Studies of baker's yeast, *Saccharomyces cerevisiae*, have helped define several important aspects of mammalian iron uptake.

The research scientists then turn the full power of modern science on to the issue of "how." Bear in mind that these distinguished scientists are with Howard Hughes Medical Institute and Division of Hematology/Oncology of Children's Hospital, Boston. The resources available to them, and the many scientists who preceded them in this field of research, are formidable. They concluded that at least seven different protein systems are known to be involved in the yeast cell transference of extracellular iron, but the most the scientists can say is that the transference process is a "hypothesis." As to the all-important issue of how the intracellular iron is transferred from within the cell to within the mitochondria, the scientists admit:

> A major site of iron utilization in the yeast cell is the mitochondrion, where iron is incorporated into heme as well as into several iron-containing components of the respiratory system. **How iron is shuttled from the**

plasma membrane to mitochondria and other sites is unknown.

"Unknown." Scientists at the Institute of Molecular Cell Biology at the University of Amsterdam reported in 1999 that **the brewer's yeast cell has at least 340 proteins "currently known to be localized in yeast," and that the processes of "translation" and the "respiratory complex" alone require "around 150 of the proteins so far known**." In other words, when a yeast cell interacts with its environment it is not a simple process. It's not a mixing of one or two chaperone proteins, it's not a pinch of a chelating compound, or a smidgeon of amino acids: it's the infinite, unknown majesty of life. It's the miracle of stepping up from inorganic molecules to the breathing moving reproducing consciousness of life. We started this section with the words of Father Teilhard de Chardin, one of the great philosopher scientists of the 20th Century. We return to de Chardin for final thoughts:

> In this cell...what we have is really the stuff of the universe reappearing once again with all its characteristics —only this time it has reached a higher rung of complexity and thus, by the same stroke...advanced still further...in consciousness.... This is the start of the living layer of our planet, the noosphere....

And this is the start of something we humans call "cultured food," which is a traditional source of nourishment for all peoples worldwide.

CHAPTER TWO

World Cultures

The use of fermentation starters might very well have its origins in the process of Euchok, the daughter of the legendary king of Woo of B.C. 4,000, known as the goddess of rice-wine in Chinese culture.... Fermentation starters are referred to as chu in Chinese, nuruk in Korean, koji in Japanese, ragi in Southeast Asian countries and bakhar ranu or marchaar (murcha) in India....
—*Fermented Cereals: A Global Perspective*
Food and Agriculture Organization of the UN, Rome 1999

The Gershwins once asked "How long has this been goin' on?" Regarding culturing, for at least 6,000 years. And that's just in Asia and India. Then there is also yogurt, wine, beer, bread, mead, kefir and on and on in the thousands of traditional foods. We are slowly coming to realize that many of these traditional foods hold great promise for the promotion of health. The World Health Organization, for example, reported in 2000 that the Japanese, with their extensive consumption of cultured soy products like miso and natto (and of course companion foods like turmeric, ginger, ocean herbs, and green tea), have the longest "healthy life expectancy" of any people on Earth. Americans, by the way, do not even break into the top 20 for healthy life expectancy. Many

Westerners are beginning to recognize that while soy or soy protein isolates are potentially anti-nutritive due to, *inter alia*, their high phytate and oxalic acid levels, cultured soy products like miso, natto, and tempeh are nutritional powerhouses with enhanced bioavailability. In India today, approximately 200,000,000 people consume daily a fermented food called "idli," and the food is so gentle and nourishing that it is regularly used in hospitals to sustain the sick and the very young. The point is simple: fermented or cultured foods have been the foundation of our world diets for what appears to be all of human history.

And we find cultured foods in places you might never suspect. Start with your morning cup of coffee. If you enjoy the rich flavors and aromas of the world's premium coffees, the "wet" processing of those premium beans involves 14 to 18 hours of fermentation by microflora such as lactic acid bacteria and beneficial yeasts. A 2001 French study in the journal *Current Microbiology* reported "throughout coffee fermentation, 60% of the simple sugars were degraded by the total microflora...." What happens is this: fermentation of the pulp breaks down complex macromolecules into simple amino acids and sugars. The original macromolecules have no flavor, but the simplified molecules have great flavor and aroma potential. The acids created in fermentation also penetrate the bean, breaking it apart from the inside and creating the compounds that explode with flavor during roasting. All the tart and fruity flavor notes of coffee are creatures of fermentation, and another result of the process is a coffee anti-oxidant profile that is most encouraging for human health. A 2001 Swiss study indicated that coffee consumption, long maligned as a vice, yields approximately four times the amount of anti-oxidants as green tea. We also adore our morning tea and its numerous confirmed health benefits, but the point is made: most of us start our day with a cup of fermented beans.

Then, as the day progresses, we may find ourselves lunching on a Reuben sandwich or some other vehicle for one of nature's healthiest foods, raw sauerkraut. Louis Pasteur waxed eloquent that raw sauerkraut was the finest vegetable food for human health, and we're sure he was referring to the rich probiotic values available from that fermented cabbage dish. Sauerkraut comes to the West from its Asian origins (a cousin of Korea's kim chee), and this food brought to Europe by invading warriors later came to be a part of the fighting rations for troops during World War I. Much like coffee, the raw cabbage of sauerkraut naturally ferments if given the right conditions. You could make your own sauerkraut by simply grinding up fresh raw cabbage, placing it into a sanitary container, and maintaining it at room temperature. A naturally present beneficial bacterium called *Leuconostoc mesenteriodes* will thrive in those conditions, creating in the process an acid environment conducive to the proliferation of lactobacilli such as *L. plantarum* and *L. brevis*. Those lactobacilli, in turn, enzymatically break down plant sugars and starches, yielding a nourishing food that is both rich in nutrients and easy to digest. Our lunch, and our health, is thus enriched by this well-traveled fermented food, praised by scientists and those who frequent refrigerated sections at natural food stores. And for those businesspeople still drinking a martini with lunch, the green olive is one of nature's most beloved fermented foods. Over 35 different strains of beneficial *Lactobacillus plantarum* have been identified in the

Spanish green olive fermentation medium.

Finally, after our morning coffee and lunch sauerkraut and olives, we deserve a little sweet confection. Enter the delicious fermented food many call "chocolate." We grow cacao on our organic farm in Costa Rica, and the fruit is sublime. And not just for us, but for the monkeys in the neighborhood, as well. The fruit is white and silky, reminiscent of a lichi, and it is a real favorite with our children. But the fruit is not the source of chocolate; rather, cocoa comes from the raw beans, which are astringent to the point of bitterness. That unpleasant bean, thick with bitter alkaloids, is also a source of food for the next generation cacao tree. Half of the weight of the bean is cocoa butter, and the rest is mostly protein and starch. On cacao plantations worldwide (and on our farm as well), workers harvest the fruit pods, cut them open, and leave them to gather airborne yeasts and bacteria. Those hungry microorganisms ferment the sweet cacao pulp, transforming bitter beans into the flavorful and anti-oxidant rich beans ready to be turned into chocolate. And if you have heartfelt thanks for the sublime flavor of chocolate, research findings from a Harvard Medical School report suggest that cocoa is naturally rich in flavenols that help to regulate blood pressure and maintain cardiovascular health. But more on that in *Chapter Three*.

This same story—raw foods fermenting into nourishing, flavorful, aromatic, easy to digest, and anti-oxidant rich foods—is repeated daily, worldwide, in literally hundreds of common foods. Appendix A to this book provides a table of many of these wholesome fermented foods, and while the list is nowhere near complete it will give you a sense of the world's reliance on cultured foods. For example, the next time you drink the cultured beverage kefir, bursting with an array of B vitamins, amino acids such as tryptophan, and the minerals calcium, phosphorus, and magnesium, recall that kefir has long been consumed by villagers of the remote Caucasus mountains and later praised by Nobel laureate Dr. Elie Metchnikoff as a foundation for longevity. In the Caucasus mountains, kefir is fermented naturally in bags made of animal hides and consumed by people legendary for long and healthy lives. You may purchase kefir today at the supermarket, but for thousands of years you would have had to enjoy it far, far away in remote mountain villages, and those villages closely guarded their probiotic recipe. Or you could enjoy another fermented milk drink, "Yakult," which may sound strange to some of you but is the world's largest functional brand of food, with over 15 million bottles of the beverage consumed daily in Japan and in many other countries worldwide. What inspired the fermented milk Yakult? The 1935 discovery by the Japanese researcher Dr. Shirota of a particularly beneficial strain of *Lactobacillus casei*, now eponymously called "*Lactobacillus Shirota*." In other words, cultured foods are everywhere on earth.

Coffee, sauerkraut, green olives, chocolate, and kefir are but a tiny representation of the cultured nourishments from the "cultures" of the world. Approximately one-third of mankind's total nourishment comes from cultured foods. One reason for the United Nation's current focus on cultured foods is that the traditional wisdom of fermentation is rapidly being lost, succumbing to forces of modernization and modern meals. This unfortunate emulation of the Western diet, with our processed foods of dubious nutritive value, is disturbing for many reasons, some of which were noted in the recent *UN Report*:

> There is a possible backlash if consumers in developing countries abandon traditional fermented foods for "smart," sophisticated products popularized in Europe and America. For example, the replacement of indigenous fermented cereal drinks with cola beverages could have a significant negative impact on daily nutrition of many consumers in developing countries. Study of traditional fermentations will undoubtedly yield new information that will expand our global knowledge of science and impact technology throughout the world.

The United Nation's report should set off alarms for those of us in the West. Seduced by "smart" and "sophisticated" products like nutritional isolates and synthetics, we run the risk of forfeiting the time-tested nutrition provided by our traditional consumption of probiotic nutrients. That risk is just as present in the aisles of vitamin stores as in mass-market America. What we lose when we eat "sophisticated" new products are the extensive medical benefits of the traditional sources of probiotic whole-food nutrition, which we next examine.

CHAPTER THREE

The Medical Benefits of Culturing

These data suggest that miso [fermented soy] consumption may be a factor producing a lower breast cancer incidence in Japanese women.
—*Nutr Cancer* 1990, Department of Nutrition
Sciences, University of Alabama, Birmingham

Butyrate, a short-chain fatty acid produced **during microbial fermentation** of fiber, induces growth arrest, differentiation, and apoptosis of colonic epithelial cells in vitro.... Thus, butyrate may reduce risk for colon cancer by inducing a pathway that enhances mitochondrial function, ultimately resulting in initiation of growth arrest and apoptosis of colonic epithelial cells.
—*Cell Growth Differ* 1997,
Albert Einstein Cancer Center, Bronx, New York

We assure you that we will begin to consider the specific nutritional benefits of probiotic vitamins and minerals, but that won't happen until *Chapters Four* and *Five*. In this chapter, we examine the process of culturing and discover how it alone confers significant health benefits. In other words, the consumption of the "growth media," the broth in which probiotics are cultured, is in and of itself highly beneficial. To borrow from a popular phrase of the 1960s, "The Medium is the Message."

Whole textbooks could be written on the health benefits of cultured soy (tempeh, miso, natto), cultured red grapes (wine), cultured milk (yogurt, kefir, Calpis, Yakult), cultured cabbage (sauerkraut) and other cultured foods, so we can do no more here than offer some highlights that will demonstrate the proven medical value of culturing. To give a frame of reference for the breadth of research on culturing and cultured foods, the National Library of Medicine contains, as of October 6, 2001, over 49,000 published references to *Saccharomyces cerevisiae* alone, just one (albeit an important one) of the host of other beneficial culturing organisms. We will thus only be skimming the surface....

A. Cancer Reduction

As the second reference at the start of this chapter from Albert Einstein Medical School reflects, the process of culturing food fiber (from whatever source, such as apple pectin) creates in the growth media a substance called butyrate. That substance, in turn, performs a vital health function in our colons: it inhibits the formation of a mischievous compound called beta-glucuronidase. Beta-glucuronidase is an enzyme that is created when pathogenic (undesirable!) bacteria rot foods like red meat in our colons, and the mischief of beta-glucuronidase is wicked indeed. Here's how it works: Our livers help detoxify our bodies and wrap up carcinogenic toxins in a kind of protective enzyme "trash bag", where the toxins can safely be eliminated from our bodies. Think of radioactive waste removal, and you get the idea. Beta-glucuronidase, however, rips open the trash bags and spills the deadly toxins back into our guts. This release of toxins is associated with colon cancer and other malignancies, so we clearly want to reduce beta-glucuronidase production. As just explained, one effective way to accomplish that is with butyrate, created in our intestines during the culturing of fiber. Note: it is not important that there are any particular vitamins or minerals present in the fiber. **The probiotic culturing of the fiber itself, without any specific nutrient assistance, creates the life-supporting compound.**

In the first reference beginning this section, the "medium" cultured was soy, and the culturing method produced the Japanese traditional food miso. The study indicated that the culturing process led to a "lower number of cancers per animal" and "a lower growth rate of cancer compared to controls." Note again, it was not that any specific nutrient was present or cultured along with the soybean paste. The cultured "medium" itself delivered the health benefit. Consider the following words of praise from Dr. Shinichiro Akizuki, director of the St. Francis Hospital in Nagasaki. From *The Book of Miso*:

> I believe that miso belongs to the highest class of medicines, those which help prevent disease and strengthen the body through continued usage....

Miso, a fermented or probiotic form of soybean, is particularly rich in genistein and daizein, both isoflavone aglycones considered to be cancer chemopreventatives. Prior to fermentation, soybeans contain "precursors" to these chemopreventatives called genistin and daidzin. It is the process of fermentation, pervasively employed with great wisdom in Japan, that converts those precursors to their active anti-cancer isoflavone form. We find it ironic that in the United States, health-conscious consumers, particularly women concerned about breast cancer, are urged to consume soy or soy protein isolates, but neither of these are the form of soy traditionally consumed in Japan. It is true that some unfermented soy—in the form of edamame—is eaten in Japan as an appetizer, but the overwhelming majority of soy consumed is in its cultured or probiotic form rich with genistein and daidzein. Our digestive systems, if populated by the right intestinal flora, can convert some of the raw genistin and daidzin into the more beneficial cancer chemopreventatives, but the low breast cancer incidence and mortality rates in Japan are clearly associated with the extensive and historic consumption of miso, natto and other probiotic soy preparations. The National Cancer Center Research Institute of Japan has, in a 2000 publication in the journal *Carcinogenesis* made it quite clear that the chemopreventative activity of fermented soy milk was at least partly attributable to the fermentation-created isoflavones genistein and daidzein, so that is the form of soy that should be consumed for maximum chemopreventative benefit.

As a final note to indicate the anti-cancer power of fermented soy, Japanese researchers at the Laboratory for Microbial Biochemistry, Hiroshima University, determined in 1993 that the cultured broth of *Saccharomyces cerevisiae* produced both bio-antimutagenic and "anticlastogenic" action in vivo and in vitro, **with mutagen formation reduced by 47%**—just from administration of the cultured broth. The "medium" was thus, on its own, a powerful inhibitor of the formation of cellular mutations. **Culturing produced unique anti-cancer "activity."**

Turning to the fascinating world of medicinal mushrooms, our respected colleague Paul Stamets wrote in his excellent book *Mycomedicinals* that the fermentation of the shiitake mushroom creates an extraordinary immune-system stimulant called arabinoxylan. Drawing upon 1995 research on ten cancer patients with advanced malignancies, Stamets reports that a compound created from the fermentation of shiitake "increased human NK [natural killer cell] activity by a factor of 5 in two months." **Culturing again creates unique compounds that stimulate powerful anti-cancer defenses.**

B. Anti-inflammatory and Anti-oxidant

Researchers at the Department of Immunology of the Bulgarian Academy of Sciences determined that the "free-radical scavenger" superoxide dismutase ("SOD") obtained from yeast cells more effectively inhibited inflammation than the SOD commercially obtained from bovine erythrocytes (cow red blood cells!). "The inhibitory effect caused by SOD [yeast] was more pronounced and strongly time- and temperature-dependent." Simply put, when you culture with *Saccharomyces cerevisiae*, as a by-product you get in the "growth media" a form of anti-oxidant SOD that is a more powerful anti-inflammatory than commercially available SOD. **Culturing produces enhanced anti-oxidant and anti-inflammatory "activity."**

The culturing of many different growth media leads to these anti-oxidant benefits. Fermented papaya, for example, is a health food preparation commonly sold in Japan. Japanese researchers in 1998 reported that fermented papaya "increased superoxide dismutase activity in the cortex and hippocampus" of animals and that it may be "prophylactic food against the age related and neurological diseases associated with free radicals." **Culturing enhances free radical scavenging.**

C. Safety and Bioavailability

Besides creating new anti-mutagenic compounds, culturing enhances the bioavailability of existing anti-mutagenic compounds in the plant. Researchers at the Department of Food Science and Nutrition, University of Minnesota, in 1995 determined that although the culturing of soy may reduce the gross amount of soy isoflavones, the resulting cultured isoflavones were significantly more utilizable by the body. Their research indicates that **culturing results in increased isoflavone "bioavailability."**

Culturing also makes food safer. Cultured soy in the form of miso is, as we've seen, a staple of the Japanese diet. Uncultured soy is unfortunately thick with an <u>anti</u>-nutrient called phytate, which seriously blocks the absorption of vital nutrients like calcium. *The UN Report* from Rome in 1999 explained that the "biotechnology" of culturing hydrolyzes phytate, and what was once an anti-nutrient, soy, now becomes a health promoting nutritious food, miso. For example, University of Alabama researchers reported in 1990 that miso supplementation led to a reduced number of cancers in treated animals and to a slower rate of growth in the cancers that did occur. As a result, the cultured miso product "may be a factor producing a lower breast cancer incidence in Japanese women." **Culturing results in enhanced nutritive value, safety, and anti-mutagenic activity.**

34

D. Cardiovascular Benefits

And, if enhanced anti-mutagenic, anti-oxidant, and anti-inflammatory effects aren't enough, culturing also creates profound cardiovascular benefits. For example, natto, created by fermenting boiled soy beans with *Bacillus natto*, contains phytonutrients that strongly inhibit the angiotensin converting enzyme ("ACE") and therefore promotes heart health. ACE inhibitors represent a significant class of pharmaceuticals, but researchers from the Tokyo University of Agriculture in 1995 confirmed that the humble boiled soy, upon culturing, did quite an effective job at the same task. **Culturing soy enhances cardioprotective activity.**

Cardiologists at a research hospital in Kyoto, Japan determined that the culturing of red grapes changed the biological activity of flavonoids. "A significant antioxidant activity was also confirmed in low-density lipoprotein from humans after ingesting red wine but not grape juice, suggesting that flavonoids in red wine can be absorbed from the intestine more efficiently than those in grape juice." **Culturing red grapes enhances cardiovascular antioxidant availability.**

The red wine research from Kyoto was confirmed in 1997 by researchers from the Université Louis Pasteur in France. Attempting to explain the "French Paradox" (the French eat a lot of fatty foods but suffer few heart attacks), the researchers determined that the culturing of red grapes changes the polyphenols in a beneficial direction. The cultured grape polyphenols show greater stability, and "since grape and wine polyphenols are chemically distinct, their antioxidant activities cannot be the same." **Culturing enhances both the cardioprotective**

"activity" and "stability" of polyphenols.

Clinical trials of Chinese red yeast rice repeatedly confirm the cholesterol-lowering benefits of that solid-fermentation product. UCLA Medical School researchers reported in 2001 that Chinese red yeast rice with appropriate levels of "monacolins" demonstrated "significant and clinically relevant cholesterol reduction." One brand of Chinese red yeast rice, Pharmanex's Cholestin, was widely respected within the medical community, and products like Cholestin and other red yeast rice ferments have the potential to reduce the risk of heart disease and thus benefit individuals and society. **Culturing rice thus also provides cardiovascular benefits.**

The fruit of the cacao tree yields, upon fermentation, the subtle flavors of cocoa and chocolate. With those subtle flavors we, the chocolate lovers of the world, get compounds called "flavenols." And research findings from Harvard Medical School strongly suggest that cocoa rich in flavenols offers strong cardiovascular protection. Harvard researchers noted that Kuna Amerinds from Central America drink an average of five cups of cocoa a day and include cocoa in many of their recipes. It is known that Kuna Amerinds do not typically have an increase in blood pressure as they age, so the Harvard researchers selected a lucky group of Boston subjects for an intensive cocoa experiment. Subjects consuming cocoa with high flavenol content experienced a healthy increase in kidney blood flow and filtering, which is consistent with the maintenance of lower blood pressure and improved cardiovascular health. We are not suggesting, of course, that people should engorge themselves with chocolate pastries and candy bars, but **the unmistakable association**

between consumption of fermented cacao seeds and cardiovascular health deserves noting.

A final note on the cholesterol-lowering effects of fermented foods. After a little chocolate, we are often tempted to drink some milk. A research review from McGill University in Canada (and several from Japan, as will be clear in the fermented milk section that follows) suggests that we wash down our chocolate with fermented milk. Writing in the *American Journal of Clinical Nutrition* in 2000, the McGill researchers eloquently summarized the relationship between fermented dairy and cholesterol reduction:

> Although not without exception, existing evidence from animal and human studies suggests a moderate cholesterol-lowering action of fermented dairy products. Mechanically, fermented milk has been shown to cause an increase in human gut bacterial content. These bacteria, once resident in the large intestine, are believed to ferment food-derived indigestible carbohydrates. Such fermentation causes increased production of short-chain fatty acids, which decreases circulatory cholesterol concentrations either by inhibiting hepatic cholesterol syntheses or by redistributing cholesterol from plasma to the liver. Furthermore, increased bacterial activity in the large intestine results in enhanced bile acid deconjugation. Deconjugated bile acids are not well absorbed by the gut mucosa and are excreted. Consequently, cholesterol, being a precursor of bile acids, is utilized to a greater extent for de novo bile acid synthesis. These actions combined are proposed as contributing mechanisms to the association of fermented milk consumption with decreased circulating cholesterol concentrations.

E. Immune Enhancement and Detoxification

We will never understand with precision how probiotics contribute to our health, but we can point to four probiotic factors that are certainly at play: Bacteriocins, Phospholipids, Beta-glucans, and Glutathione.

Bacteriocins

The Law of the Jungle also applies to our microscopic friends, and probiotics compete against "unfriendly" flora by creating natural antibiotics. Called "bacteriocins," these heat-stable proteins deposited in the growth media literally destroy closely related pathogenic bacteria, much to our gratitude. It seems that probiotics don't like to be crowded, especially by distant weird cousins who might overstay their welcome and eat their food supply. In just one *Lactobacillus plantarum* strain responsible for green olive fermentation, for example, **Spanish researchers** determined the probiotic "was able to produce bacteriocins throughout the incubation period (15 days)." Spanish researchers also turned their lab benches into barstools and examined the bacteriocin activity of lactic acid bacteria in Rioja red wine. The researchers located 42 strains of lactic acid bacteria in the red wine, nine of which (all *L. plantarum species*) demonstrated antimicrobial activity. **Nigerian researchers** obtained ten bacteriocin-producing compounds from three Nigerian fermented foods (kenkey, ogi, and wara), and the research determined that "the bacteriocinogenic properties of the local isolates of *Lactobacillus* can help to reduce hygienic risk and the spoilage of fermented foods." Mukumbi, a traditional **Zimbabwean** wine made from fermented mapfura fruit, is not hospitable to toxic *salmonella* and *shigella*. The unfermented fruit is quickly populated by those dangerous pathogens, but the fermentation process has rapid antimicrobial action according to 1999 research at the University of Zimbabwe. **Turkish researchers** determined that "tarhana," a fermented yogurt-cereal mixture that is a dietary staple of Turkey, contains organic acids that retard spoilage and inhibit pathogens. This dramatic bacteriocin capability is confirmed again and again in the scientific literature; indeed, in the National Library of Medicine there are, as of November, 2001, over 4,400 references to published scientific papers on these bacteriocins. Research published in the *American Journal of Clinical Nutrition* in 2001 gives a sense of how valuable these probiotic allies can be:

> Premenopausal women have a flora of mostly lactobacilli, and certain properties of these strains, including adhesive ability and production of acids, bacterocins, hydrogen peroxide, and biosurfactants, appear **important in conferring protection to the host.**

Clemson University researchers in 1993 similarly described the protective role of probiotic bacteriocins in dairy fermentation:

> During growth in fermented products, dairy starters, including lactobacilli, lactococci, leuconostocs, streptococci, and proprionibacteria, produce inhibitory metabolites. Inhibitors include broad-spectrum antagonists, organic acids, diacetyl, and hydrogen peroxide. **Some starters also produce bacteriocins or bactericidal proteins active against species that usually are related closely to the producer culture.**

The Special Effects Against Candida Albicans

Candida infections, truly a pervasive scourge, deserve special consideration. Recent research indicates "Candida infections were decreased during yogurt consumption regardless of the presence of live or heat-killed bacteria." This highlights our previous point that the "Medium is the Message," as it is not necessarily the presence of live culture that leads to the beneficial effect—the antifungal effect is instead achieved from the compounds created in the growth medium. Many people, unfortunately, deprive themselves of the candidicidal (Candida killing) benefits of probiotics such as those in yogurt, fearing that all microorganisms are somehow bad and may promote Candida overgrowth. This unfounded fear is particularly acute in the case of *Saccharomyces cerevisiae*, or Brewer's yeast, for many people equate Brewer's yeast with its wholly dissimilar and distant relative *Candida albicans*. Those strains of yeast, far from being alike or cooperative, are in fact highly competitive and antagonistic, and the science is quite clear that when *Saccharomyces cerevisiae* are cultivated, they create powerful candidicides that would help control or prevent Candida yeast infections. For example, a Japanese study in 1986 demonstrated that the acidic fraction of a *Saccharomyces cerevisiae* culture exerted a "significant protective effect against *Candida albicans* infections...." Additionally, it is known and we have explored how *Saccharomyces cerevisiae* strengthens a person's immune system through the creation of beta-glucans and other culturing by-products, which stimulate "host defense" against all fungal and other pathogenic infections. Moreover, Candida infections can lead to a particular vitamin "biotin" deficiency leading to skin disorders. Culturing with *Saccharomyces cerevisiae*, conversely, creates highly bioavailable and nourishing biotin, thus directly responding to a common Candida symptom.

Finally, we offer an image to aid in the understanding that Brewer's yeast is NOT an unwelcome yeast. Visualize poison ivy and spinach leaves. One leaf is toxic, another delightfully nourishing and beneficial. They are both plants and both have green leaves, but that's where the similarities end. So, too, with *Saccharomyces cerevisiae* and *Candida albicans*: both are yeasts, and both are tiny, but that's where the similarities end.

Phospholipids

There is considerable attention now being given to other compounds produced by probiotics called phospholipids for their enhancement of human liver functioning. Biochemist Paris Kidd writes in his article "Phosphatidyl Choline: A Superior Protectant Against Liver Damage" that phosphatidyl choline benefited all human subjects in a large-scale clinic in Germany. The phospholipid helped reverse or improve conditions ranging from liver fatty degeneration to all stages of inflammation and fibrotic damage. Yeast cells, the "mini-mammals" that they are, produce considerable quantities of beneficial phospholipids that are available during the consumption of fermented media. For example, in 2001 the *European Journal of Biochemistry* published research from the Institut für Biochemie in Austria as follows:

> Large parts of the endoplasmic reticulum of the yeast, *Saccharomyces cerevisiae*, are located close to

intracellular organelles, i.e. mitochondria and the plasma membrane.... This plasma membrane associated membrane (PAM) is characterized by its high capacity to synthesize phosphatidylserine and phosphatidylinositol.

The same research institute published findings in 1988 that depict a similar process:

> Like other yeast cellular membranes the outer mitochondrial membrane contains predominantly phosphatidylcholine (44% of total phospholipids), phosphatidylethanolamine (34%) and phosphatidylinositol (14%).

Long words for a simple point: **Culturing creates highly beneficial phospholipids that are available through the consumption of cultured media and that support enhanced liver functioning.**

Beta-glucans

Beta-glucans are also major components of yeast cell walls that have profound biological activity. Beta-glucan supplementation is strongly associated with increasing the activity of the immune system and reducing elevated cholesterol. Research on yeast-cultured beta-glucans is ongoing, and there is promise that beta-glucans from yeast will play an important role in complementary medicine. For example, a research report in 2001 from the Harvard Medical School highlights the value of dietary consumption of beta-glucans from yeast:

> Heart disease is the leading cause of death in the U.S. One way to reduce the risk of developing the disease is to lower serum cholesterol levels by making dietary

changes. **In addition to reducing intake of total fat, and dietary cholesterol, serum cholesterol can be further reduced by added fiber, especially from sources rich in beta-glucan…. The yeast-derived fiber is a more concentrated source of beta-glucan than the oat product.** It is currently being tested in a wide variety of food products.

Culturing with *Saccharomyces cerevisiae* provides a concentrated form of immune and cardioprotective beta-glucans.

Detoxifying Glutathione

The ability to adapt and respond to chemicals and toxins in the environment is fundamental to all life forms, and probiotic nutrients enhance our crucial detoxification capabilities. The world is on fire with smoke, pollution, and chemical assaults, and our cells—and the cells of probiotic organisms—have evolved defense systems against chemical insult. One key aspect of our cellular defense is a compound called glutathione, and it performs much the same function in *Saccharomyces cerevisiae* as it does in human life. Researchers in Japan cultured *Saccharomyces cerevisiae* in a medium rich with the amino acids comprising glutathione, and the brewer's yeast cells were able to metabolize the isolated chemicals and thus increase the levels of their intracellular glutathione. The researchers performed a series of tests on these enriched yeast cells, and the research results "strongly suggest that intracellular glutathione plays an important role in the adaptive response in *S. cerevisiae* to oxidative damage." **Accordingly, consuming *Saccharomyces cerevisiae* may provide a supplemental source of glutathione and aid**

in the detoxification of chemical toxins.

F. A Special Focus on Fermented Milk

Now back to yogurt and other fermented milk foods. *The Danone World* Newsletter provides an excellent scientific resource on the medical value of yogurt. In the July 2001 issue, the article "Fermented Milk and Successful Ageing" offers an elegant summary of some of the research on this all-important source of probiotic nutrients:

> Diet is one of the most important factors influencing the complex processes of ageing. Fermented milk has its place in the dietary prevention of age-related disorders. With regard to nutrition, fermented milk helps to maintain food and water intake, which are often reduced in older people. With regard to health, the beneficial effects of fermented milk against osteoporosis and impaired lactose digestion have now been clearly demonstrated. Encouraging early results suggest that fermented milk has a positive effect on the immune defense system, intestinal transit, muscle mass and cardiovascular disease. Other avenues that merit investigation include colon cancer and cataract.

Research from Japan and New Zealand confirms another important health benefit of cultured milk consumption: enhancement of immune system function. From the Juntendo University School of Medicine in Tokyo, research on nine healthy human subjects demonstrated that **drinking fermented milk for three weeks led to a significant increase in the subject's natural killer cell activity**, and this increased immune-system functioning "remained elevated for the next three weeks."

From New Zealand in 2001, a report was published stating that dietary consumption of **"fermented foods such as yogurt...can enhance production of Type I and Type II interferons at the systemic level"** and reduce the development of allergies.

Oregon State University reported in 1996 that yogurt consumption is correlated, epidemiologically, with a reduced risk of colon cancer. The University researchers determined that **the anti-mutagenic effect from yogurt was not due to the presence of live active culture but on the anti-mutagenic compounds produced during fermentation.** From Milan, Italy researchers confirmed that yogurt has shown anti-tumor activity against colon and breast cancer. Once again, **the scientists determined that the activity was not from the living bacilli but from the compounds created during the culturing process.** "The antiproliferative effect was not related to the presence of bacteria in fermented milk." From the *American Journal of Clinical Nutrition* in 2001, researchers at the Federal Research Centre for Nutrition in Germany highlighted the superior anti-mutagenic value of the culturing media:

> Notably, some of our newer studies showed that short-lived metabolite mixtures isolated from milk that was fermented with strains of *Lactobacillus bulgaricus* and *Streptococcus thermophilus* are more effective in deactivating etiologic risk factors of colon carcinogenesis than are cellular components of microorganisms.

In other words, compounds created by fermentation in the milk have greater anti-cancer effectiveness than the naked cells of the probiotics themselves.

Where There's a Will, There's a Whey

As we've just explained, it's not just the live probiotics in yogurt that have health benefits but also the compounds created in the fermentation of yogurt. For example, French researchers recognized that a healthy probiotic ecology (in simple terms, lots of friendly gut flora!) in the colon was associated with a reduction of beta-glucuronidase. In turn, reducing beta-glucuronidase is associated with a reduced risk of colon cancer. You will recall that beta-glucuronidase is the enzyme created by pathogenic bacteria fermenting foods like red meat. The research from France is highly significant, for it demonstrates that a person can eat a food that will promote exceptional health benefits and strongly promote the growth of beneficial intestinal flora. And that food? It is the whey created in the process of the fermentation of milk. The researchers determined that simply giving the human subjects whey formed during the fermentation of milk was sufficient to change intestinal pH, lower beta glucuronidase levels, and increase the strength of already existing intestinal flora. **Culturing thus creates unique pre-biotic nutrients, apart from the viable bacteria, that promote the growth of beneficial bacteria, the health of the digestive system and reduce the risks of colon cancer**.

It is crucial to always bear in mind that while many of the benefits of fermented products may derive from the presence of "viable" or living probiotics in the food, **the key point of this chapter is "The Medium is the Message."** Even when the fermented foods are pasteurized or otherwise do not deliver live culture, many important health benefits have been scientifically confirmed. A Symposium on "Probiotic Bacteria: Implications for Human Health" was recently published in *The Journal of Nutrition*, and beautifully illustrates this point. For the 50 million Americans diagnosed with **hypertension**, the Symposium observed that "bioactive peptides resulting from the proteolytic action of probiotic bacteria on casein (milk protein) during milk fermentation may suppress the blood pressure of hypertensive individuals." When *Saccharomyces cerevisiae* and *L. helveticus* ferment milk, two "tripeptide" by-products "function as angiotensin-I-converting enzyme ("ACE") inhibitors and reduce blood pressure." Indeed, a Japanese company has developed a "pasteurized" fermented milk product (Calpis) based on this line of research, and the symposium correctly notes that for this Japanese product, "the effect is mediated by a fermentation end product, not viable cells themselves." A human clinical trial on thirty elderly hypertensive patients demonstrated that taking Calpis fermented milk for eight weeks successfully reduced both systolic and diastolic blood pressure. In a related animal study, hypertensive rats were given Calpis, and within **six hours** their abdominal aorta levels of angiotensin I-converting enzyme was "significantly lower." The data from this study also demonstrated that the ACE inhibiting peptides in the Calpis fermented milk "**are absorbed directly without being decomposed by digestive enzymes**, reach the abdominal aorta, inhibit the angiotensin I-converting enzyme, and show antihypertensive effects in spontaneously hypertensive rats." We believe these compounds are being absorbed "directly" without interference, due to their probiotic predigestion and enhanced stability due to culturing co-factors. In a placebo controlled human clinical trial on 28 hypertension patients, cell wall fragments of *L. casei* were administered orally and small "but significant" decreases in systolic pressure, diastolic pressure, and heart rate were observed. From McGill University in Canada, research published in the *American Journal of Clinical Nutrition* in 2001 similarly noted the "association of fermented milk consumption with decreased circulating cholesterol concentrations." From Tel Aviv University and Ben Gurion University in Israel, scientists determined in an animal study that byproducts of *Lactobacillus bulgarius* fermentation provided long-term cardioprotective benefits and significantly improved "functional recovery" after a heart attack. Simply put, heart tissue was saved and restored to viable functioning, and life was prolonged. **By-products of culturing lower blood pressure and thus aid in the treatment of hypertension and elevated cholesterol, and protect against death from heart attacks.**

The Probiotic Bacteria Symposium was called to praise live culture, not to bury it, so the focus on the "end products" of culturing should not be misinterpreted. Indeed, one of the most prized features of the Japanese fermented milk Yakult, the world's largest functional food brand, is that science has confirmed that its *Lactobacillus casei* strain "Shirota" exhibits such excellent survival in the gastrointestinal tract. There is thus great value to yogurt, kefir, Yakult and other fermented milk drinks that deliver live active culture, but the Symposium sounded the clear message that the "Medium is the Message" —

The literature suggests several situations in which viability is not required for some activities. Improved digestion of lactose…, some immune system modulation…, and antihypertensive effects…have been linked to nonviable cells (cell components, enzyme activities or fermentation products.)

Culturing in and of itself, apart from any vitamin or mineral enhancement, apart even from the presence of live active culture in the food, creates nutrients (see Appendix B) that are of extraordinary value in promoting health. Upon that foundation, it is now time to explore the positive relationship between cultured foods and specific nutrients. As a segue to the next sections, consider the following conclusion of researchers from the Department of Microbiology at the University of Texas:

> It is apparent that one or another of the lactic acid bacteria requires each of the B vitamins required by animals and assay methods developed during study of nutrition of bacteria and yeasts have played a large role in the initial or independent discovery, isolation, and characterization of vitamins, vitamin derivatives, and functionally similar substances. Clear examples include biotin, biocytin, lipoic acid, nicotinic acid, pantothenic acid, pantetheine, folic acid and tetrahydrofolic acid (and their derivatives, pyridoxal, pyridoxamine, and pyridoxamine phosphate).

As we stated in the beginning of this paper, these microorganisms are a bridge between the inorganic and life. We will fully cross over the Life Bridge in *Chapter Five*, but first we will define our terms in *Chapter Four* so we can share a scientific language and speak without confusion about this most confusing topic. In *Chapter Four*, we will expose the terms "USP," "Isolates," "Mixtures," and "Probitoic Nutrients" to sunlight, and see which ones actually grow.

PROBIOTIC FACTS

"...It is documented that our Palaeolithic forefathers not only consumed millions of times more LAB (lactic acid bacteria), but also several times more fruit and vegetable fibres. Furthermore, the selection of plants eaten was significantly larger. It is suggested that they ate an average from approximately 500 plant species, which gave the humans of that time a much larger variation in the prebiotics supplied, and consequently a wider production of various synbiotics. This larger variation in plant consumption compared with that of today facilitated the greater availability of a larger amount of the more than two million chemical compounds that constitute the human body. It may or may not be a coincidence that increases in inflammatory conditions in general, allergic conditions, obesity, coronary heart disease, and cancers in the western world have paralleled the decreased consumption of probiotics and prebiotics, but also a reduced variation in the prebiotics consumed."

"...It is likely that several hundred thousand, if not millions, of synbiotic compounds are released by microbial fermentation, and are subsequently absorbed. Among these are various short chain and other fatty acids, amino acids, peptides, polyamins, carbohydrates, vitamins, and numerous antioxidants and phytosterols [7]. More than 4000 plant flavonoids have been identified, approximately 600 carotenoids, and some of these have an antioxidant potential 10 times as strong as that of vitamins C and E."

"...Genetically greater differences are observed between LAB than between fishes and humans."

"...the most pronounced effects seem to be achieved through the use of mixtures of several probiotic LAB...probably in combination with several prebiotic fibres...."

—*Curr Opin Clin Nutr Metab Care* 2001;4(6):571-9. Pre-, pro- and synbiotics. Bengmark S. Department of Hepatology and Surgery, University College of London, Liver Institute. PubMed UI: 11706296

CHAPTER FOUR

USP, Isolates, Mixtures, and Probiotic Nutrients:
A Glossary of Commonly Misunderstood and Misapplied Terms

> Why, you might just as well say that 'I see what I eat' is the same thing as 'I eat what I see'!
> —The Mad Hatter, *Alice in Wonderland*

The Mad Hatter's confusion about backwards and forwards language is a common problem in the "natural" products industry. Everything under the sun seems to call itself "natural," and the term is so regularly applied "backwards and forwards" that it's lost meaning. For example, we would all agree that walnuts and garlic grown in selenium-rich earth are naturally rich in organic selenium. We, of course, eat such foods with pleasure. But does the selenium isolated and extracted from those foods also qualify as "natural"? And is the selenium mineral isolated from rocks or soil also just as natural for human consumption? If so, then the word "natural" has no real meaning for humans, for no human in history has ever eaten a meal of isolated selenium or a nice pulverized rock.

We thus discard the term "natural," and using supplemental selenium as an example, let's together create a useful "glossary" that will guide us throughout this book:

A. "USP" Elements.

USP of course refers to the United States Pharmacopoeia, and the USP forms of the mineral include "selenite" and "selenomethionine." Such mineral or molecular forms are emphatically "not food." They are perhaps better described as "homeless molecules," separated from their cellular homes and identities. Consider, for example, a Material Safety Data Sheet description of the hazards of sodium selenite, a common and inexpensive USP form of selenium used in many vitamin supplements:

> **POISON! DANGER! MAY BE FATAL IF SWALLOWED. HARMFUL IF INHALED. CAUSES SEVERE IRRITATION TO SKIN AND EYES. CAUSES IRRITATION TO RESPIRATORY TRACT. AFFECTS LIVER, KIDNEYS, BLOOD, SPLEEN.**

> **A proper label for USP sodium selenite should proceed to warn that a person should not get the chemical "in eyes, skin, or on clothing," and that "if swallowed, induce vomiting immediately…. In all cases, get medical attention immediately."**

We think all would agree that while such a potentially poisonous chemical is "naturally" present in the earth, it doesn't qualify as a natural "food." The Devil is always in the dosage, and there will be those who argue that an appropriate, and presumably minute, amount of the pure chemical sodium selenite is good for you. On the other hand, there is disturbing research that indicates that selenite, if taken in high dosages, may create pro-oxidative stress on human DNA. For example, in April, 2001, the Texas Tech University Health Sciences Center reported that:

> Because the public may frequently supplement [selenium] compounds at high dosages, the possible pro-oxidative effect of [selenium] becomes a concern.... Our laboratory has shown previously that high dosages of SeL [selenite] resulted in cytotoxicity and induction of 8-hydroxydeoxyguanosine (8-OhdG) in DNA of primary human keratinocytes....

The marker compound 8-OhdG is indicative of pro-oxidative stress on DNA, precisely the opposite effect of that sought by those taking selenium supplements. Accordingly, it is important to understand that while there are advocates for selenite supplementation, we will demonstrate that it acts on (or against) the body in a manner different from selenium obtained from food.

B. "Isolates."

Selenomethionine is another USP form of selenium, but it differs from sodium selenite in that it is an isolate obtained from food. For example, selenomethionine (commonly refered to as SeMet) is significantly present in some wheat gluten and in brewer's yeast grown in a selenium-enriched environment ("selenium yeast.") It is a step in the direction of a whole food, but it is to whole food what soy protein isolate is to soy, curcumin is to turmeric, or caffeine is to green tea. In other words, it is just one chemical, albeit organic, isolated from its complex organic plant origins.

C. Mixtures of USP forms with other foods ("Mixtures")

If you add a USP form of selenium to other foods, you have just that: a "mixture" or what some call a food-based product. When consumers eat a breakfast cereal enriched with USP selenium, they consume a "mixture" of the mineral with foods. If you add a few flower petals to a gallon of USP chemicals, what you have is USP chemicals with a few flower petals. And let's not delude ourselves: if you add four milligrams of acerola cherry to 300 milligrams of ascorbic acid, what you have is a chemical with a whisper of a hint of an echo of a trace amount of a whole food. But that highway mirage of whole food does not, in our opinion, justify putting pictures of cherries and oranges on the label and calling the product "natural." Then there is one company adding USP vitamins and minerals to fast-food burritos, and virtually every glass of milk or processed orange juice contains vitamin and mineral fortification. Or you could start your day with a bowl of mass-market breakfast cereal and get 100% of a person's daily requirements for chalk ("calcium carbonate"), add some enriched bread or soy milk, and pretty soon you're a chalk holding tank, ready for any blackboard that passes by. Some companies mix USP compounds with other isolates, like isolated proteins or amino acids, on the theory that such a mixture is more than the sum of the isolated parts. Many companies offer Mixtures of varying forms.

D. Probiotic Nutrients

The United States Department of Agriculture in June, 2001 reported that certain whole foods contain significant quantities of organic selenium, specifically identifying wheat gluten and commercial selenium yeast. **The NIH Clinical Center's "Facts About Dietary Supplements" notes in accord that plants grown in soil or an environment rich in selenium create "the major dietary sources of selenium in most countries throughout the world."** In other words, consumers don't have to obtain supplemental selenium in either USP, Isolated, or Mixture form: people can successfully obtain selenium in organic form from whole and cultured whole foods.

Let's digress for one moment from the building of the "glossary" to consider the importance of this mineral nutrient in our diet. We will return to selenium in *Chapter Five*, but a quick look at the nutrient demonstrates its health significance.

According to the NIH Clinical Center report on supplemental selenium, a selenium deficiency is commonly associated with increased AIDS mortality, the enlarged heart and poor heart function in Keshan Disease, thyroid dysfunction, exacerbated neurological damage from iodine deficiency, and rheumatoid arthritis. Just as there are dangers associated with too little dietary selenium, there are recognized profound benefits from increased "whole food" selenium. In a major study underwritten by the NIH and the American Cancer Society and published in 1996 in the *Journal of the American Medical Association*, probiotic selenium in the form of selenium yeast was given to 1312 patients during the period 1983-1991.

> **Over the course of 8,271 "person years," the selenium yeast treatment resulted in "significant**

reductions in total cancer mortality...total cancer incidence...and incidences of lung [46%lower risk], colorectal [58% lower risk], and prostate cancers [63% lower risk]. Primarily because of the apparent reductions in total cancer mortality and total cancer incidence in the selenium group, the blinded phase of the trial was stopped early. No cases of selenium toxicity occurred."

In 1999, published research from Kansai University in Osaka, Japan compared the bioavailability of selenium yeast versus sodium selenite. After examining both the accumulation of selenium in tissue and the beneficial anti-oxidant activity of glutathione peroxidase, the researchers concluded that **selenium "in SeY [selenium yeast] is more bioavailable than selenite Se, and therefore it is the preferred form for supplementation."**

Researchers from the Arizona Cancer Center and the Arizona College of Public Health are conducting continuing research on the anti-cancer properties of selenium yeast. As reported in the journal *Urology* in April, 2001, the supplemental use of **"selenium in selenized yeast decreased prostate cancer risk by almost 60%."**

In perhaps the most compelling evidence of the profound difference between probiotic selenium and USP or purified selenium, the journal *Science News* reported in April, 2001 that "rats getting the purified selenium additives (selenomethionine or selenocysteine) had 50% more [precancerous colonic] aberrant crypts than did rats getting selenium as part of the broccoli they ate." The lead researcher, Dr. John Finley of the Human Nutrition Research Center, concluded elegantly that "**[s]omething in the whole food must boost selenium's anti-cancer property.**"

There is also something refreshing in such an honest admission that we just don't know everything about the infinite complexity of nature.

There are a number of sources of whole food selenium. As mentioned above, whole food selenium is present in foods grown in a selenium-rich environment, and includes foods like brazil nuts and walnuts. Probiotic whole-food selenium, or selenium yeast, is also available from a number of sources. One product, SelenoMax® from Nutrition 21, was used in the NIH/University of Arizona study published in *JAMA*. The Institut Roselle in Canada also manufactures and supports research on this important anti-cancer probiotic nutrient. Another probiotic or yeast-grown selenium is offered by New Chapter, Inc. (see Appendix C). **In research conducted in 2001 at the University of Scranton by Dr. Joseph Vinson, one of the world's leading antioxidant researchers, New Chapter's probiotic selenium yeast was found to have 64 times the anti-oxidative power of Selenomethionine**.

Comparison of Antioxidant Quality

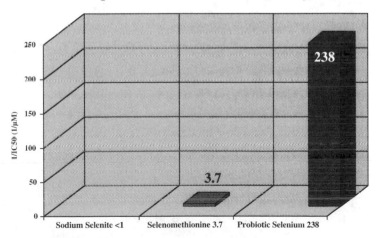

There is thus healing power in the whole food that laboratory synthetics cannot replicate. This all-important point was perhaps best expressed by nutritional expert Paul Pitchford in his brilliant work *Healing With Whole Foods*:

> Vitamins within plants and living organisms are organized into extremely subtle and complex patterns composed of many other nutrients. Such patterns cannot be duplicated except in a living environment. Thus, vitamins in whole food are often immeasurably more effective than the synthetic variety: furthermore, the lifeforce in whole foods is absent in synthetic vitamins.

The "glossary" is now complete, and it permits us to share a vocabulary as we proceed to examine the relative merits of the various forms of vitamin and mineral supplements. We have already expressed our clear conviction that supplementation with the living complexity of probiotic foods is preferable to the recent experimental use of purified or isolated nutrients. No one has better expressed this perspective than Nobel laureate Albert Von Szent-Gyorgyi, M.D., the discoverer of ascorbic acid:

> The deeper we go into the facets of life, the more mysteries we encounter. Analyzing living systems, we often have to pull them to pieces, decompose complex biological happenings into simple reactions. The smaller and simpler the system we study, the more it will satisfy the rules of physics and chemistry, the more we will understand it, but also the less 'alive' it will be. So when we have broken down living systems to molecules and analyzed their behavior, we may kid ourselves into believing that we know what life is, forgetting that molecules have no life at all.

CHAPTER FIVE

The Life Bridge of Probiotic Nutrients

Let your food be your medicine, and your medicine be
your food.
　—Hippocrates

We look to Hippocrates as the founder of our medical
tradition. He was correct: our food can be our medicine,
and should also be the preferred source of our nutritional
needs. Let's review the evidence in support of the
wisdom of probiotic nutrients:

A. Selenium

We developed our glossary by referring to the various
forms of supplemental selenium, and our revisiting of
selenium will be brief. First, it is absolutely settled that
Saccharomyces cerevisiae can metabolize and incorporate inorganic selenium into their cellular tissue. A recent
published study from the Technical University of Budapest
summarized the research on this point:

> Selenium (Se) is an essential micronutrient for human
> and animal organisms. Organic selenium complexes
> and selenium-containing amino acids are considered the
> most bioavailable. Under appropriate conditions yeasts

are capable of accumulating large amounts of trace elements, such as selenium, and incorporating them into organic compounds.

Previously, researchers in Finland published in 1986 their simple statement of the power of brewer's (also known as baker's) yeast (*Saccharomyces cerevisiae)* to transform the "inorganic" into the "organic":

> Baker's yeast is able to assimilate carbon, nitrogen, phosphorus and sulphur sources together with a great number of minerals and trace elements into a palatable, nutritious product. The metabolism of yeast is precisely controlled during the production growth phase and thus it is possible to determine the composition of the product by controlling the raw materials…. **Analysis of the protein fraction of selenium yeast has shown that selenium is present in all the major soluble proteins**.

This assimilation of the inorganic into the organic, this alchemical transformation of the lifeless into life, is the miracle of probiotic nutrients. *Saccharomyces cerevisiae* **and other probiotics thus become a "life bridge" between the world of molecules and the world of man**.

The procedures for such selenium yeast culturing are not obscure or controversial. As recently as 1999 the Department of Food Science and Human Nutrition of Iowa State University published its "protocol for incorporation of sodium selenite or sodium selenate into *Saccharomyces cerevisiae* by continuous fermentation…." As we stated above, it is our understanding that companies such as Nutrition 21, the Institut Rossell, and New Chapter utilize the yeast culturing of selenium to achieve this organic probiotic form of the nutrient.

There is also no question that the probiotic nutrient form is highly preferable to the potentially more toxic inorganic form. Research previously cited from the National Cancer Institute demonstrated that selenium yeast reduced all forms of cancer mortality by 50%, and the Arizona Cancer Center reported that selenium yeast reduced the incidence of prostate cancer by 60%. This is consistent with prior research from the Division of Nutritional Sciences at Cornell University, which reported in 1987 that selenium yeast supplementation was associated with "reductions in total cancer mortality and in the incidences of lung, colorectal, prostate and total cancers."

Two animal studies further illuminate how selenium yeast is preferable to the inorganic forms of selenium supplementation. Researchers from the Swedish University of Agricultural Sciences gave sodium selenite or selenium yeast to two sets of nursing dams. The selenium status of their respective calves was then assessed, and the nutritional distinction was dramatic:

> The Se status of the calves in the selenite group was considered to be marginal, but the status of the calves in the yeast group was considered to be adequate. Supplementation of the suckler cows' diet with organic Se in the form of Se yeast rather than sodium selenite improved the Se status of their calves.

Follow-up research at the Swedish University considered selenium supplementation for "growing" cows. The heifers were fed no supplementary selenium for six months. After that depletion period, the heifers were divided into four groups. Group I received sodium selenite, Group II sodium selenate, Group III selenium yeast, and Group IV was the control. The researchers concluded that the "concentration of selenium in blood and plasma was significantly higher in group III than in groups I and II, but there was no significant difference between groups I and II." In other words, the "inorganic" forms were roughly comparable, but supplementation with probiotic selenium was superior.

Hungarian research on giving human infants supplemental selenium is also highly instructive. At the National Institute of Rheumatology and Physiotherapy in Budapest, scientists noted that <u>for adults</u> selenium yeast demonstrated higher intestinal absorption and bioavailability. These scientists investigated the effect of probiotic selenium on pre-term infants living in low selenium areas in Hungary. One group of pre-term infants was given supplemental probiotic selenium, and the control received no form of selenium. After just two weeks, the serum selenium levels of the supplemented group showed material improvement, while the control group demonstrated measurable decline. The researchers concluded:

> Compared with previous studies, our results suggest that the bioavailability of selenium in the form of yeast selenium is higher than that of other selenium compounds used for preterm infants. We did not observe any complications or side-effects owing to enteral yeast selenium supplementation. We conclude that selenium enriched yeast is a safe and an effective form of short-term enteral selenium supplementation for infants.

The medical case for the probiotic form of selenium is conclusive.

B. Iron and Copper

We address iron and copper together because of the intimacy of their intracellular relationship. Both minerals are present in all body tissues, and have indispensable roles in the formation of hemoglobin and collagen. Iron and copper are used by the body to maintain fatty acid oxidative balance, and both are involved in the production of noradrenalin (stress response hormone). Iron is also a key co-factor in the production of serotonin and dopamine (neurotransmitters), and copper is necessary for proper bone formation and the production of RNA.

Much of what science understands about the human absorption and utilization of iron and copper come from the study of *Saccharomyces cerevisiae*. Researchers at the Howard Hughes Medical Institute explained in 1999 that "studies of yeast iron transport" inform our understanding of mammalian transmembrane iron transport. Regarding copper transport within yeast cells, research demonstrates:

> Studies with yeast cells have revealed that several proteins are used to pick up copper ions, as they are transported from the outside environment through the inside of the cell, and to shuttle them to appropriate copper metalloproteins. These shuttles, or 'taxicabs,' have proteins having names such as Atx1, Lsy7, Cox17, and CCC. **Each of these proteins have a human equivalent**. For example, the human equivalent of the yeast's CCC is the human Wilson's protein....

The close relatedness of yeast and human copper transport led the scientists to a lovely moment of near-poetry:

> One should take interest in attempts to predict human physiology from studies with yeast. Although one might hesitate to call yeasts "mini-mammals," the field of yeast genetics has provided us with much of our knowledge of how human cells work.

We, of course, agree, hence our description of such probiotics as the "Life Bridge" between the inorganic and human physiologies. We understand from these "mini-mammals" that at least six proteins are responsible for the transport of extracellular iron into the yeast cells, and that it is still "unknown" precisely how this is accomplished. We know that there is a delicate dance between the transport of iron and copper into the Brewer's yeast, and that an iron deficiency "necessarily accompanies copper deficiency." As a result, scientists have discovered that there is "transcriptional cross-talk between the iron and copper metabolic pathways," and this extends to the "major transcriptional regulator of yeast copper metabolism." **Simply put, a Brewer's yeast cell senses the presence of iron and copper in its environment, computes its intracellular requirements, uses an intricate and ever-shifting array of metabolic pathways and proteins to incorporate the needed amounts of those minerals in the correct ratios, and that these processes, still not fully understood, are also occurring in human cells.**

It is no surprise, therefore, to learn that many laboratories and companies are culturing iron and copper to enhance their human bioavailability and suitability. Iron in an elemental form is potentially toxic and pro-oxidative, but without iron we can develop anemia and perish.

Copper in an elemental form is a pro-oxidant, but when organically bound by yeast metabolism the pro-oxidant becomes, according to recent research from Dr. Joseph Vinson of the University of Scranton, an anti-oxidant. Dr. Vinson explains "this may be due to the fact that the cupric ion is not free, i.e. in an organically bound form. Binding of a metal ion can change its oxidative potential." Dr. Vinson also determines that probiotic iron exhibits materially less potential pro-oxidative effect than the inorganic iron. Dr. Vinson's research was conducted on the iron and copper organic yeasts from New Chapter, and it is our understanding that the Institut Roselle is also conducting research and product development on probiotic iron and copper yeasts. This is the glory of taking compounds potentially toxic in their isolated states and rendering them suitable and beneficial for human nutrition through culturing.

There is wide consensus that the culturing of food creates a desirable form of these metals. When iron is cultured by yeast, for example, "heme" is created, which is the most assimilable food form of the compound. The use of soy as the culturing medium is also advantageous, for iron is naturally present in soy. Culturing soy also enhances iron bioavailability, for the fermentation of soy activates phytase, an enzyme that neutralizes the iron absorption inhibition of phytate. The use of culturing biotechnology for iron and copper thus has confirmed scientific validity, and it delivers the nutrients in their most advantageous form.

C. Chromium

Chromium is considered essential for maintenance of
normal glucose tolerance, and a chromium complex
occurring in brewer's yeast, termed glucose tolerance
factor (GTF), was found to be of outstanding quality.
—Nippon Rinsho 1996 Jan;54(1):79-84 Department of
    Biochemistry, Faculty of Medicine, Tottori University

There is wide consensus that chromium yeast, especially
in the form of GTF chromium, is the ideal nutritional
source of chromium.   During culturing, *Saccharomyces
cerevisiae* incorporates chromium ions into their cells.
Scientists at the Laboratory of Fermentation and Yeast
Technology, University of Zagreb, noted in 2001 that chromium ions became bonded to protein molecules in yeast,
and that GTF was also generated during fermentation. It
sounds simple, but it isn't.

In the *Journal of Inorganic Biochemistry*, scientists
reported that their laboratory was able to separate "eleven
apparently homogeneous chromium-containing fractions
from a brewer's yeast extract." Four of the fractions
contained no GTF, one had a "slight degree" of GTF
activity, four other fractions showed "varying degrees of
GTF activity," and two were deemed "biologically
inactive," which means simply that the scientists couldn't
figure out what they did. In other words, GTF, so needed
by today's Syndrome X'ers and incipient diabetics, is all
over the yeast cell, in multiple forms, and no one really
knows whether they all have to be present to work or if
one is the pharmaceutical "silver bullet." What we do
know is that the yeast cell and enzyme systems closely
resemble human cells, and if the yeast cells need to put

chromium in at least eleven places, who are we to say that only one form is biologically meaningful.

To compound the mystery of Glucose Tolerance Factor, research from France throws the entire chromium-GTF relationship into question. The scientists duly noted the discovery of GTF in 1957, and observed that most of the studies on GTF have used brewer's yeast as the starting material. There was a "presumption," the researchers state, that the "active" material in GTF is a "complex" containing chromium ions. That was the accepted wisdom, but it didn't bear out in research. In what was surely a surprise finding to many scientists,

> [i]ndividual fractions with GTF activity did not differ between Cr-rich and Cr-deficient yeast, and there was no relationship between Cr content and GTF activity. This does not support the hypothesis that chromium is an obligatory constituent of the GTF, assuming that GTF is a unique substance.

If one were to provide chromium in a USP, Isolate, or Mixed form, which ion of chromium should thus be chosen to maximize the delivery of usable GTF? Or better yet, which of the eleven organic forms of chromium present in the yeast "mini-mammal" should be isolated to best promote the formation of GTF? Or better yet, which of the five GTF-chromium variants is the best to isolate? Or better yet, is GTF related to elemental chromium at all? The world's scientists have struggled to answer those questions, but the answer lies somewhere within the mystery of living whole food. Fortunately, probiotic GTF-chromium is available, and is clearly the preferential form of the nutrient.

D. Coenzyme Q-10

> Though an old man, I am a young gardener.
> —Thomas Jefferson

That is a pleasant goal: to be old in years, but young at heart and connected to the physical joys of nature. The problem is our bodies sometimes fail, our muscles and immune system ache for oxygen, and we succumb. One important factor in that demise is the diminishing supply of a quasi-vitamin sometimes called Vitamin Q, or more commonly COQ-10.

The scientific term for the quasi-vitamin is "coenzyme ubiquinone," referring in part to its "ubiquitous" role in human physiology. The term "coenzyme" means simply that the compound is used by the body to make an enzyme function, and in this case COQ-10 facilitates the functioning of at least three mitochondrial enzymes. These enzymes are involved in the production of adenosine triphosphate (ATP), the currency of energy sustaining all cellular functions. The Nobel Prize was awarded in 1978 for research on the biological transfer of energy, which in part turned on the "proton-motive" role of COQ-10 in energy transfers. We are not dealing with a trifle here, but a profound survival component needed to sustain life.

There is promising research from countries around the world (Japan, United States, Sweden, Italy, Germany) demonstrating that COQ-10 supplementation improves cellular energy and cardiovascular functioning, and thus helps to reverse the severity of cardiovascular disease. This is not surprising given the striking concentration of COQ-10 in heart tissue. The National Cancer Institute is now suggesting that COQ-10 supplementation may invigorate the immune system and has a role to play in a complementary response to breast cancer. Scientists in Sweden have led research on COQ-10's role as an anti-oxidant and free radical scavenger. Persons with end-stage AIDS demonstrate a severe COQ-10 deficiency, which clearly would compromise the activity of their immune systems. In other words, COQ-10 is a serious and critical compound.

In 1958, a research team from Merck determined the chemical structure of COQ-10 and produced it via **fermentation**. COQ-10 is also available as a USP supplement, but it is present in a number of foods, most notably from a brewer's yeast culture. Impressive research from the laboratory of Dr. Joe Vinson of the University of Scranton once again confirms that the probiotic form of the vitamin nutrient, created for New Chapter, is superior to its USP analog. In research completed in April of 2000, Dr. Vinson determined that probiotic COQ-10 yeast was more stable and exhibited twenty times the anti-oxidative quality and effectiveness compared to a USP version.

Concentration of CoQ10 to Inhibit LDL and NLDL

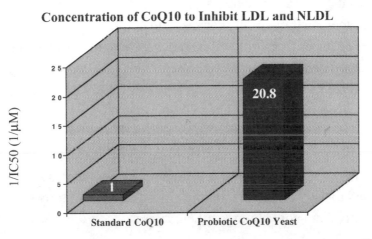

Remember: when Dr. Vinson analyzed the probiotic COQ-10, it was in its probiotic medium as part of whole food. In other words, the COQ-10 was exerting its antioxidative effect together with the cultured soy and the antioxidants created by the combined activity of *Saccharomyces cerevisiae* and multiple beneficial bacteria. It's thus almost not a fair comparison, for the "naked" isolate of COQ-10 could not possibly bring to bear the exquisite array of living antioxidants created in the culturing of whole food.

That additional potency is impressive to us, but perhaps in a way far different than you think. The typical reaction to hearing about a supplement's (or pain killer's, or anti-inflammatory's) superior potency and bioactivity is "now I can take the same dosage and get even more effect." We think that is a serious and all too common mistake. The goal with all supplementation should be "less is more," and the less we deviate from traditional approaches to nourishment, the better. Human health is, after all, based on an endless gentle rhythm of eating wholesome foods, digesting them properly, and gaining balanced nourishment. All of life, in turn, is based on the deeper rhythms of proper rest and activity. It's a matter of balance. Too little water, and we die from dehydration. Too much water, and we drown. Too few calories, and we die of malnutrition. Too many calories, and we die of morbid obesity. Too little Vitamin A, and we suffer neurological damage. Too much Vitamin A, and we suffer precisely the same neurological damage. Too little Vitamin C, and our antioxidant deficit can lead to athero-sclerosis. Too much Vitamin C, and it may turn pro-oxi-dative and contribute to atherosclerosis.

Scientists have a term for this: biphasic. One phase or level of food or drug consumption is healthy, and at a higher phase of consumption the same substance causes injury. Children might call this "The Goldilocks Effect." Too little of a nutrient is damaging, too much is just as damaging, but then there is the "just right" amount that Goldilocks was seeking. That's what an intelligent supplement program also strives to achieve, so when we learn from Dr. Vinson's work that probiotic COQ-10 yeast exhibits twenty times the antioxidant power of USP COQ-10, that is an opportunity to **reduce** our intake of the supplement, even though it's in the form of beneficial probiotic whole food. We just don't want to take too much of anything, for "less is more."

We are reminded of the writings of the wise gardening essayist, Henry Mitchell. Mr. Mitchell for many years wrote the "Earthman" column for the *Washington Post*, and he was inspirational for his humble and humorous insights. When asked to reflect on the key lessons of a lifetime of gardening, he wrote:

> The most valuable of all lessons for the gardener is that if we are not quite sure what we are doing (which is almost all the time) it is infinitely better to do nothing than to guess.

We are humble in the face of all that we do not yet understand about the human body. Like Henry Mitchell, who spent a lifetime learning that he didn't know anything "for sure" about gardening, we feel comfortable advising our patients and readers to take a balanced, conservative, and safe approach to almost everything, including their nutritional programs. What we know "for sure" is that humans have safely derived nourishment from probiotic whole foods for millennia. When Dr. Vinson's research indicates probiotic COQ-10 is a more powerful anti-oxidant, that is consistent with our scientific judgment that food works better (and differently) in our body than chemicals. It also tells us to "garden safely," and allow a lower and biologically reasonable dosage of probiotic COQ-10 to work with the body. And then take time to smell the flowers....

E. Vitamin C

Industrial-scale production of ascorbic acid also starts with glucose. The sugar is first reduced to sorbitol and then oxidized with Acetobactor suboxidans to L-sorbose. The diisopropylidene derivative of the latter is oxidized to the corresponding derivative of the L-2-ketogulonic acid. After removal of the protecting isopropylidene groups, L-ascorbic acid (Vitamin C) is obtained via L-2-ketogulonic acid.

—H.D. Belitz & W. Grosch, *Food Chemistry*

ASCORBIC ACID SYNTHESIS

Glucose

▼

Reduction to Sorbitol

▼

Oxidation to L-Sorbose

▼

L-Sorbose diisopropylidene oxidation

▼

Corresponding derivative L-2-ketogulonic acid

▼

Removal of protecting isopropylidene groups

▼

Ascorbic acid

This is what the natural products industry calls Vitamin C. It is impossible for you to have ever eaten an L-ascorbic acid berry, for it is plainly not a whole food. In fact, the compound is dramatically more refined than white table sugar, being a distant chemical descendent of glucose. We are not condemning the chemical compound, but it is important to have a clear picture of the industry's most popular anti-oxidant vitamin. An ester (chemical fusion) of ascorbic acid and calcium carbonate (chalk) is also widely available under a number of brand names, and there are Mixtures that compound ascorbic acid with a variety of other materials.

There are also a number of whole food sources of Vitamin C. Freshly picked blackberries, strawberries, raspberries, acerola cherries, a number of fruits and melons, and raw probiotic cabbage (aka sauerkraut) contain "meaningful" amounts of Vitamin C. Probiotic Vitamin C is also available, much like the probiotic coenzyme Q (COQ-10), iron, selenium, and the other nutrients we've been exploring. Probiotic Vitamin C will, depending on the formulation, deliver up to 250 mg of Vitamin C per dosage.

How is Vitamin C Biosynthesized?

The mechanisms used by *Saccharomyces cerevisiae* to biosynthesize and incorporate Vitamin C, just as with other nutrients we've considered, remain largely cloaked in the mystery of whole food. After all, how does a blackberry do it? With respect to brewer's yeast, scientists describe it as a "mini-mammal," for it shares many cellular features with human life and other mammals. Curiously, it does not share with humans the ability to biosynthesize Vitamin C, for humans and other primates have lost the ascorbate biosynthesis capability. In other words, yeasts, plants, and many mammals can synthesize Vitamin C, and human life thus depends on these allies for this all-important antioxidant. But how these allies biosynthesize Vitamin C is a complex process that we are just beginning to understand.

We do know for a fact, however, that brewer's yeast and probiotic bacteria do biosynthesize many vitamins and coenzymes like COQ-10 and Coenzyme A. There are some "The Earth is Flat" people who refuse to acknowledge that yeast has a broad range of vitamin synthesizing capabilities, but we respectfully disagree. For example, we know, for a fact, that the intracellular Vitamin D receptor (VDR) process for humans exhibits a "similar pattern" to the VDR in brewer's yeast. Research published in 1993 in the journal *Molecular Endocrinology* illustrates the close connection between yeast and human vitamin metabolism: "The mechanism for VDR up-regulation is conserved in both yeast and mammalian cells."

The probiotic synthesis of Coenzyme A also reveals the extraordinarily complex processes undertaken by "Life Bridge" allies to synthesize these nutrients:

Coenzyme A is biosynthesized by bacteria in nine steps. The biosynthesis begins with the decarboxylation of aspartate to give beta-alanine. Pantoic acid is formed by the hydroxymethylation of alpho-ketoisovalerate followed by reduction. These intermediates are then condensed to give patothenic acid. Phosphorylation of pantothenic acid followed by condensation with cysteine and decarboxylation gives 4'-phosphopante-theine. Adenylation and phosphorylation of 4'-phoshopantetheine completes the process.

We do know, within the limits of science, that yeast cells biosynthesize ascorbate to protect their tissue from oxidative damage. Vitamin C, for humans, is part of our "extracellular"—or outside the cell wall—response to free radicals that can create oxidative damage. That's why Vitamin C is recommended to help us prevent the oxidation of LDL and other blood lipids, for those are extra-cellular, or beyond our cell membranes. **But, once again, how do yeast cells biosynthesize and use ascorbate**?

Science is giving us only glimpses, and it's by no means a complete picture. *Saccharomyces cerevisiae*, like the more complex life forms it resembles, has an elaborate array of defenses to extra-cellular free radical damage. In a 1998 study reported in the *Journal of Biochemical Chemistry*, scientists noted that *Saccharomyces cerevisiae* "has at least 14 proteins that participate in ROS [reactive oxygen species, including free radicals] protection. This recent study observed that ascorbate (Vitamin C) is useful for free radical protection outside the cell wall, but that it is not useful "within the plasma membrane." It is no surprise that the yeast cells thus evolved an enzyme system that stabilizes the ascorbate and allows it to participate in the defense of the cell wall. How is this done? Scientists have some interesting theories about the role of compounds such as Coenzyme Q6 in the yeast plasma membrane, but that is largely irrelevant. The simple point, made by those scientists in the 1998 report, is "extracellular ascorbate stabilization is an activity present not only in yeast but in other animal and plant cells." **Somehow, using at least 14 proteins and other enzymes and co-factors, ascorbate becomes part of the yeast cell's defenses**.

To further illustrate the almost infinite complexity of this living process, researchers from the University of Exeter wrote, in 2001:

> Biosynthesis of L-ascorbate (vitamin C) occurs by different pathways in plants and animals.... Yeast synthesizes D-erythroascorbate from D-arabinose and D-arabinono-1,4-lactone in a pathway analogous to that in plants. The plant, mammalian, and yeast aldonolactone oxidase/dehydrogenases that catalyze the last step in each pathway have significant sequence homology.... **Assessment of the literature reveals that little is known about many of the enzymes involved in ascorbate biosynthesis or about the factors controlling flux through the pathways.**

In other words, the biosynthesis of ascorbate happens, it happens in brewer's yeast cells, it is created in a living form, but we don't know precisely how. And that's a perfectly comfortable position for those of us who rely on living plants and "Life Bridge" allies to provide this nutrient, for it is on **their** innate intelligence that we can safely depend. The mischief comes when people **think** they know how nature creates a living nutrient, and they attempt to throw some ascorbate, amino acids, and protein chaperones into a pot, mix it all together and proclaim: "This is life." In our humble opinion, we think not. It is, we deeply feel, a Dr. Frankenstein vanity to posture even for an instant that humans know how yeasts or other probiotics accomplish the miracle of life.

What we as humans can do, and do regularly, is use "Life Bridge" allies to biosynthesize ascorbate and other precious living compounds. Much like using bacteria to create yogurt, penicillin, or other antibiotics, or yeasts to create wine and bread, we can structure controlled conditions where "Life Bridge" allies can be encouraged to biosynthesize living nutrients. **And now we'll share with you a key fact that we've been reserving for just this moment: Within the vitamin manufacturing industry, many vitamins are manufactured either exclusively or increasingly by probiotic processes.** This was observed by researchers at the University of Ghent in Belgium, 1992, who in their article "Microbial Production of Vitamins and Biofactors: An Overview" noted "Recently, an increased implementation of biotechnological fermentation and bioconversion processes is noticed in the vitamin industry." We all need to savor that observation: although the vitamin industry has for years relied on organic chemical synthesis, it is now a "trend" for vitamins to be probiotically cultured.

This "trend" is clearly present for a host of hitherto "chemically synthesized" vitamins. As the faculty at the University of Ghent observed:

> However, for several of these compounds (for B-carotene, vitamin E, vitamin F-group), microalgal culture procedures… and/or microbiological processes (for vitamins K2, B1, B5, B6, B8) rapidly emerge and some are already competing with the existing chemical processes, especially the microalgal derived fat-soluble vitamins: provitamin A, vitamin E and the PUFA'S.

The report is even more emphatic (encouraging) with respect to the fermentation production of other vitamins:

> **Other vitamins and related biofactors are now produced exclusively via fermentation**: ergocalciterol

(D2), riboflavin (B2), cyanocobalamin (B12), orotic acid (B13), vitamin F-group (also via extraction), ATP, nucleosides and coenzymes (NAD, NADP, FAD, coenzyme A and Q, adenosyl-methionine (Ado-met), L-adenosyl-homocysteine....Vitamin C is produced via a combination of chemical reactions and one fermentation step.

Consistent with the report from the University of Ghent, we understand that a major USP manufacturer of ascorbic acid is considering a complete shift from inorganic synthesis of Vitamin C. **And that is precisely what is occurring throughout the vitamin industry**. Again, as noted by the faculty of the University of Ghent, after the vitamin industry, either exclusively or increasingly, probiotically cultures our essential vitamins, the purified "USP" form is isolated out of the living food or probiotic culturing media. How is this isolation accomplished? Well, it evidently is not simple, for just as the culturing of the nutrients is cloaked in living mystery, "the recovery and purification of these vitamin compounds from their fermentation broth is equally complex." This is the bitter irony of the vitamin industry: it uses "Life Bridge" organisms to create our vitamins, those living nutrients are infused with the healing power of traditionally cultured foods, and then the miracle of life is thrown away in order to deliver the vitamins in a chemically purified form. Some day, when we as a society can look back at this brief experimentation with USP and isolated nutrients, we suspect that scientists will shake their heads in disbelief....

Returning to Vitamin C, we of course recommend that people always choose the whole over the part, thus the ideal source of Vitamin C would be either probiotic Vitamin C or fresh organic fruits and vegetables naturally rich in Vitamin C.

The Lesson of Goldilocks

Now we turn to another aspect of the Vitamin C story. In the prior section on COQ-10, we introduced the concept of "biphasic" nutrition. The problem of "too little" or "too much" is solved by the "just right" amount of nutrients available from a whole food. There is perhaps no better example of the biphasic nature of vitamin consumption than the case of Vitamin C. In the United States and the United Kingdom, the RDA for Vitamin C remains a conservative 60 milligrams per day. By contrast, believers of the Orthomolecular Theory contend that humans need to take thousands of milligrams of synthetic ascorbic acid in order to maintain health. Because of some early high profile advocates of this theory (such as Linus Pauling), many people became religious about Vitamin C use and started taking 2,000 or more milligrams of the chemical. Not of the "food," but of the chemical cousin of glucose more refined than table sugar.

People took it as received wisdom that mega-potencies of Vitamin C were good for you, and it was heresy to question that belief. Not any longer. In 1998, British researchers from the University of Leicester reported that although the consumption of 500 mg of ascorbic acid did, on one level, reduce oxidative stress, on another level "there was a deleterious effect superimposed on that." That deleterious effect was an **elevation in a blood marker indicating DNA oxidative damage**. From the University of Minnesota Medical School in 1991 came a consistent report that at "physiologic" levels (at or under the RDA) ascorbate acted as an anti-oxidant, but at "pharmacological" levels the chemical acted as a pro-oxidant. A study presented in 2000 at the American Heart Association raised additional alarms, for people taking "just" 500 mg of ascorbic acid appeared to be hastening the onset of hardening of the arteries. More recent research from the University of Pennsylvania indicated that even 200 mg of ascorbic acid could trigger DNA oxidative damage. All of these studies have been attacked by the Orthomolecular "true believers," as would be expected. These studies are a direct assault on the value and safety of taking huge quantities of ascorbic acid, but we don't pretend to be able to resolve the controversy in this book. For those of us who embrace the probiotic approach to vitamin supplementation, our "dog is not in that fight." Perhaps, in the fullness of time, after generations of use and study, scientists will determine that humans need to take mega-potencies of refined or synthesized ascorbic acid, either on its own or estered with chalk. Maybe. Maybe not. Until then, we can resort to the tried and true method of obtaining our nourishment from whole and probiotic foods.

A postscript: in the aftermath of all the contention about the possible damaging effects of high dosages of ascorbic acid, there are some notable "reexaminations" of earlier positions. Dr. Andrew Weil, whose scholarship and leadership we profoundly admire, once endorsed the 1,000-2,000 mg per day blanket recommendations. No longer. In 1999, he noted on his website that the *Journal of the American Medical Association* in April, 1999 reported that "200 mg a day is the maximum human cells

can absorb, making anything above that level a waste."
He went on to cite another study, this time (ironically)
from the Linus Pauling Institute itself, which "identified
a similar dose, 120 to 200 mg, as the optimal amount for
reducing the risk of cardiovascular disease, cancer,
cataracts and other chronic conditions." We are delighted
to see that distinguished leaders in the field of
complementary medicine are revisiting the issue of
mega-potency dosages of ascorbic acid. It takes courage
to challenge the old "USP" paradigm, but in our
judgment it is time for a return to the safe and reasonable
nutrition available from cultured whole food.

Now, a final and perhaps controversial point on the
"bi-phasic" nature of ascorbic acid. Vitamin C in the form
of USP ascorbic acid (straight up, estered or "Mixed") is
one of the most popular dietary supplements, and the overwhelming majority of consumers take pharmacological
dosages of this compound. Without even thinking much
about it, consumers will **on a daily basis** take 500-1,000
mg of ascorbic acid, and such consumers are subjecting
their physiologies to many times the body's normal
physiological capacity of that USP isolate. That does not
strike us as reasonable, but consumers are encouraged to
do so by advertisements and labels that suggest that the
pharmacological dosages are nothing more than
concentrated grapefruits, cherries or oranges. Those
advertisements play into the bizarre mindset of modern
supplement takers who are convinced that "more" is
invariably "better." These same consumers will,
however, carefully select only the freshest organic
produce that has never seen a chemical on its soil, but
then think nothing of going into the vitamin aisle and

popping mega-potencies of USP compounds many times more refined than white sugar. It's almost a split personality within the natural products industry, and we frankly don't buy into it.

We are not, however, <u>universally</u> condemning a mega-potency dosage of USP ascorbic acid; rather we reject giving a consumer a pharmacological dosage of a highly refined substance willy-nilly, <u>in all cases</u>, in light of the potentially bi-phasic nature of Vitamin C. To us, if a pharmacological dosage of Vitamin C in its USP form is ever to be used, it should be with the cautious mindfulness that it is for discrete and limited use, such as with any drug, and certainly under the supervision of a health care practitioner. Conversely, we believe that people should regularly enjoy a lower potency of Vitamin C from whole or probiotic food.

F. Calcium

> This shortly brought them to a bewitching spring, whose basin was incrusted with a frostwork of glittering crystals; it was in the midst of a cavern whose walls were supported by many fantastic pillars which had been formed by the joining of great stalactites and stalagmites together, the result of the ceaseless waterdrip of centuries.
> —Mark Twain, *The Adventures of Tom Sawyer*

Have you ever tried to imagine how Tom Sawyer and Becky Thatcher felt when they first came upon the "fantastic pillars" of the limestone cave? If so, and if their sense of bewildered wonderment has evaded you, we have a recommendation: go to your nearest grocery store, travel down the vitamin aisle, and there before you will appear a modern-day limestone cavern. In other words, you will have entered the "calcium section."

Why is the calcium section a "limestone cavern?" Because a great number of the calcium supplements are simply ground up and pressed limestone, otherwise known as calcium carbonate or chalk. Other USP or Mixed forms of calcium take that calcium carbonate and flavor it, mix it with amino acids, dress it up with chelates and chaperones, play with its molecular form, or otherwise manipulate it. There are also more inventive chemical variations on the calcium theme, but those basically still offer the "glittering crystals" of calcium in one form or another. And then there are the most adventurous calcium supplements that will grind up seashells. Unless you're an otter, we suspect seashells were never on your family's dinner table – to eat that is. Simply put, most of the calcium supplements you will find today are not food.

There are, however, some that are. One from a major producer of nutritional supplements in the natural products industry recently caught our attention. This interesting formulation offers a probiotic fermentation of organic soy (itself a great idea), and the product literature further states "Calcium, added during fermentation, is converted to the soluble lactate form, thereby improving absorption." We haven't studied the fermentation process used to create this product, but the concept seems wholly appropriate. It appears to deliver a probiotic form of calcium, which seems to be an intelligent alternative to the USP or Mixed forms.

New Chapter also has a probiotic whole-food calcium/magnesium formulation, which fulfills our requirement that the nutrients be provided in a whole food form. New Chapter's Cal/Mag combination offers 75 mg of probiotic Calcium, 75 mg of probiotic Magnesium, and a supporting cast of whole food minerals and herbal extracts. We are comfortable with the reasonable potency of this formulation, and both of the foregoing probiotic calcium supplements appear consistent with the 1999 study reported in the *International Journal of Food Sciences and Nutrition*, which demonstrated that the fermentation and germination of foodstuffs contribute to the enhanced bioavailability of calcium.

But there will be consumers who enter the "limestone cavern" seeking much higher potencies of calcium than offered by either of the above probiotic products. More often than not, such consumers will have a fixed notion that they must supplement their diets with at least 1,000 mg of calcium per day or risk accelerated bone loss. It's a terrible fear that motivates these consumers, and we appreciate their anxiety. They have seen the many tragedies of osteoporosis: hip and femur fractures, immobility, and the loss of freedom of movement. People want to grow old but still, like Thomas Jefferson, enjoy the splendors of the garden. They are afraid of nursing homes and wheelchairs, and if to avoid those it means taking "glittering crystals" of inorganic limestone, or ground up seashells, so be it. But we respectfully disagree, and offer what we think is a more sensible nutritional concept. Our concept is called "food."

Let's study the "theory" of mega-potencies of calcium. It is based on a simple syllogism: Bones are made of calcium (and many other minerals as well, in living tissue). As people age, they lose bone mass. Therefore, giving people huge quantities of elemental calcium will avert or reverse bone loss. That theory is revered as "Truth" in many quarters, but does it stand up to scientific examination? Let us take the heretical position and say, "we do not believe so," and it's important to briefly challenge the theory. It won't take long....

The Three Little Pigs

First, we need to understand that bone mass doesn't mean bone strength. It's simply part of the "theory's" syllogism that massive means strong, but consider: a house can be built of a massive amount of straw, or a slender amount of brick. Ask the Three Little Pigs which house turned out to be stronger. It's not the mass; rather, it's the **strength**, the resistance to fracture, that is key. And that's where the syllogism starts to crumble. There is evidence that high consumption of calcium is associated with **increased** bone fractures. From the University of Sydney comes the study, reported in the *American Journal of Epidemiology*, of over 9,700 white women from the United States. These women completed a "validated food frequency questionnaire," and data on new non-vertebral fractures were collected every four months over a mean follow-up period of 6.6 years. Vertebral fracture data were based on spinal radiographs done a mean of 3.7 years apart. In other words, this study was rich with data, and it drew the following conclusions:

> There were no important associations between dietary calcium intake and the risk of any of the fractures studied. **Current use of calcium supplements was associated with increased risk of hip...and**

vertebral...fractures; current use of Tums® antacid tablets was associated with increased risk of fractures of the proximal humerus....

Professor Colin Campbell, a nutritional biochemist at Cornell University, was the subject of an extensive article in the August, 2000 issue of *Discover Magazine*. Dr. Campbell has devoted a lifetime of study to the theoretical association between calcium consumption and bone fracture, and the article reports:

By the 1990's, nutrition researchers had gathered data from different parts of the world and found another surprising correlation: **The more calcium people consumed, the more susceptible they seemed to be to hip fractures.** People in those countries that consume the highest levels of dairy foods (North American and northern European nations) take in two or three times more calcium yet break two or three times more bones than people with the lowest calcium intake (Asians and Africans).

As to Asians, Dr. Campbell further noted that:

Most Chinese were getting their calcium from vegetables and fruits alone. Although they got less than half the calcium recommended by the USDA, their bones seemed healthy. Among women over 50, the hip fracture rate appeared to be one fifth as high as Western nations.

Lest anyone quibble that the above data pertains to non-white, non-Americans, the Harvard Nurses' Health Study should silence the skeptics. In that 12-year study involving 78,000 nurses, the nurses reported on their consumption of dairy foods, and data were collected on arm and hip fractures. The Harvard researchers noted a correlation:

> **Nurses who drank the most milk—two or more glasses per day—broke more bones than the others**. They had a slightly higher risk of arm fracture (1.05 times) and significantly higher risk of hip fracture (1.45 times).

The "mega-potency" syllogism may be worshipped as "Received Wisdom" and "Truth," but it clearly doesn't correlate to the experience of cultures around the world. As succinctly stated by the *Journal of Postgraduate Medicine* in 1978, there are societies that have virtually no osteoporosis whose women consume as little as 250 mg of dietary calcium. Dumping more "straw" on top of the Little Pig's house won't make it any stronger: in fact, evidence supports the opposite conclusion.

If mega-dosages of elemental calcium don't help, can they hurt? The first step in answering that is determining how much of the supplemental calcium is actually absorbed. According to research from Creighton University School of Medicine published in the *Journal of Bone Mineral Research*, the answer is not much. The research considered 189 middle-aged women in good general health, and they were subjected to 526 absorption studies over a 17-year period of observation. The finding: "There was a highly significant inverse correlation between calcium intake and absorption fraction." Sounding a bit like a high-school geometry class, the scientists explained "the absorption fraction is approximately inversely proportional to the square root of intake." Simply put, the more calcium the women consumed, the more they **didn't** absorb. At low intakes of calcium, the women absorbed approximately 45%, but at intakes above 2000 mg/day they absorbed approximately 15%. Worse yet, as the women aged, there was a "highly significant fall in absorption efficiency."

Where is all this unused, unabsorbed calcium going? Not only is supplemental calcium consumption NOT adequately correlated to bone strength and reduced bone fractures, and not only do women appear to lose the capacity to absorb the calcium as their intakes and age increase, but what happens to all this "glittering crystal" of limestone that people are dumping down their gullets? We suppose that the best case is that people have sufficient digestive and detoxifying capability to rid themselves of the excess, but it seems tragic that we force people to use up their body's detox resources in responding to supplemental calcium. And that's the best case....

The Big Bad Wolf

There is disturbing evidence that an excess of supplemental calcium may be correlated to a number of disease conditions.

- **Cardiovascular Problems:** *The Journal of Cardiology* reported in 1991 that the need for calcium is greatly reduced in old age. There is thus a potential hazard that in old age a small amount of calcium may find its way into the body's soft tissues. The aorta is notably prone, resulting in the loss of elasticity. In addition, the journal *Calcified Tissue International* reported that a variant of calcium crystals called calcium hydroxyapatite may induce formation of liposome aggregates that are a step in atherosclerotic plaque calcification. In a 1993 issue of that journal, researchers reported that cholesterol and calcium phosphate "accumulate in atherosclerotic lesions."

• **Arthritis:** In a variety of joint diseases apatite crystals have been identified as a principal constituent. In the *Annals of Internal Medicine*, researchers observed "Other crystals causing arthritis have also been identified, including calcium...[and] calcium hydroxyapatite crystals." Crystal-induced arthritis is "characterized by acute articular inflammation...."

• **Kidney Stones:** Researchers at the Harvard School of Public Health reported in 1997 "High intake of dietary calcium appears to reduce risk for symptomatic kidney stones, whereas intake of supplemental calcium may increase risk." This research abstract thus confirms what should be obvious: mineral crystals are not food, and the body reacts differently to the differing sources of calcium.

• **Prostate Cancer:** *Reuter's* reported on September 28, 2001 that there appears to be an elevated risk of prostate cancer for men who consume more than 600 mg of calcium from dairy products. Dr. June Chan of Harvard University led the research published in the

American Journal of Clinical Nutrition, and in the group of nearly 21,000 men studied, those who consumed more than the 600 mg of calcium from dairy products had a 32% higher risk of prostate cancer than men who consumed no more than 150 mg of calcium a day. Dr. Chan sounded the following sensible caution:

> While we would like to see additional confirmatory studies, men taking calcium supplements may wish to reassess their need for calcium supplements and perhaps discuss their individual risk-benefit tradeoffs with their physicians given their health history.

These examples are not meant to alarm, but to highlight the inherent risk of taking mega-potencies of a chemical in excess of the body's capacity or need. The body needs reasonable amounts of dietary and probiotic calcium, a balanced amount of exercise, fresh air, sunlight, and rest, and there are also herbs and spices that play an important role in preserving bone integrity. We should resort to these time-tested and moderate strategies, and not lose ourselves in the limestone caverns.

G. Vitamin B

> Changes in the vitamin content of cereals with fermentation vary according to the fermentation process, and the raw material used in the fermentation. **B group vitamins generally show an increase on fermentation**.
> —"Fermented Cereals: A Global Perspective"
> *FAO Bulletin No. 138*, United Nations, Rome 1999

We decided to conclude our exploration of probiotic nutrients with the B group, as it is frankly the least intellectually strenuous and most enjoyable probiotic vitamin to consider. After all the scientific detail on Vitamin C, calcium, selenium and the others we have explored, we all deserve an easy stroll, a victory lap, and the B vitamins are just that. And with our victory lap, we think traditional societies would approve of a nice dark Dopplebock beer to fulfill our vitamin B needs.

Vitamin B needs from beer, you ask? Just consider:

> This style of beer (Dopplebock) is traditionally associated with Lent.... Because the [Bavarian monks of St. Francis of Paula] cut down on their eating during Lent, they needed to get their nutrients in some other fashion. In 1634 they came up with a special Lenten beer called Paulaner Salvator, in honor of the Savior who would rise on Easter. Because Dopplebock had to take the place of bread for over six weeks, it was especially rich in nutrients, including folate and vitamin B-6, as well as antioxidants.
> —*The Schlafly Growler*, The Saint Louis Brewery and Tap Room, Volume 7, Issue 2, Feb. 2001

We suspect that the fasting monks also enjoyed one of the prime functions of the B complex vitamins, which is to maintain the normal activity of the nervous system. The B vitamins certainly also aided the monks during their lengthy sessions of prayer and meditation, for the vitamins provide the body with energy by aiding in the conversion of carbohydrates to glucose. And speaking of conversions, the B complex vitamins are commonly referred to as coenzymes because they help our enzymes carry out thousands of molecular conversions in the body.

But enough of monks, conversions, and beer…

This section is the triumphant moment for one of our favorite probiotic allies, *Saccharomyces cerevisiae*, or "Brewer's Yeast." The process of fermentation, both outside and inside our bodies, is one of the principle sources of all the B vitamins. First, let's look "outside" the body.

In Indonesia, a cultured soy food called "tempeh" is a staple of the diet. Soybeans, like many plants and vegetables, are naturally low in vitamin B-12, containing less than one ng (nannogram) of B-12 per gram of raw soy. In a research report from the Journal of *Applied Environmental Microbiology,* 1977, we find that after inoculation of the soy with the bacterium common to tempeh, the culturing produced 148 ng. of B-12 per gram. **In other words, there was a 148 times increase in Vitamin B-12 via the bacterial fermentation of tempeh**.

Saccharomyces cerevisiae (or Brewer's Yeast, during this Victory Lap) has a broad ability to biosynthesize the B vitamins. In 1997, Wayne State University researchers noted "**the yeast *Saccharomyces cerevisiae* has been shown to be an excellent model system in which to understand the regulation of inositol metabolism**." Those researchers, writing in the Journal of *Molecular Microbiology,* 1997, observed that Brewer's Yeast growing "in the presence of inositol" (in other words, isolated **inositol** was part of growth medium) showed an increase in an associated enzyme. Notably, this "in vivo" enzymatic reaction did not occur "in vitro," so something in the **living** yeast was conscious of its environment, and was able to bring the "inorganic" to life. We see here another expression of the genius of the "Life Bridge."

Researchers from Spain in 1995 determined that Brewer's Yeast catalyzed the formation of **riboflavin** from a precursor chemical. Italian researchers in 1998 demonstrated that **Brewer's Yeast mitochondria can "take up externally added riboflavin and synthesize" two separate flavin nucleotides**. Researchers from the Polish National Academy of Sciences in 1997 located the yeast gene responsible for the biosynthesis of **nicotinic acid**. Not surprisingly, this Brewer's Yeast gene is "homologous" to the corresponding human gene responsible for the biosynthesis of this folic acid.

Japanese researchers in 2000 outlined the biosynthetic pathways of **thiamin**, and demonstrated that Brewer's Yeast could synthesize thiamine (**Vitamin B-1**) "under both anaerobic and aerobic conditions." **Researchers from Germany determined that eleven different proteins, working in specific sequence, are involved in the uptake of thiamin into the Brewer's Yeast**. This 1998 research also confirmed that Brewer's Yeast "utilized external thiamin for the production of thiamin diphosphate (ThDP) or can synthesize the cofactor itself." Once again, the "Life Bridge" organisms have the ability to interact with their growth medium—their environment—and determine how to create the organic out of the inorganic.

Researchers in Canada determined that chicks fed probiotic Vitamin **B-6** fared significantly better than with isolated Vitamin B-6 alone. In fact, removing the Brewer's Yeast "provoked a severe symptomatic deficiency." **The B-6 nutrients in the context of Brewer's yeast were thus significantly more bioavailable**.

As touched upon in our prior discussion of Vitamin C, Brewer's Yeast cells have the ability to biosynthesize **pantothenic acid (B-5)**. Researchers from Du Pont Pharmaceuticals in 2001 observed that "contrary to previous reports, Brewer's Yeast is naturally capable of pantothenic acid biosynthesis." If you hadn't realized that was in scientific question, it was. And it's crucial, for with biosynthesized pantothenic acid the Brewer's Yeast is able to biosynthesize Coenzyme A, critical to the Brewer's Yeast (and human) cell's breakdown of fatty acids.

Other "Life Bridge" allies have important roles to play in the biosynthesis of B vitamins. For example, researchers from the Department of Microbiology and Immunology at the University of Kentucky reported in 1993:

> *Lactobacillus plantarum* requires **biotin** for growth. **We show that in the presence of high levels of the biotin biosynthetic precursor, dethiobiotin,** *L. plantarum* **synthesizes biotin** and grows in medium with dethiobiotin but without biotin. *Lactobacillus casei* also grew under similar conditions.

We thus have "Life Bridge" allies working on the <u>outside</u>, but some are welcome allies working to create B vitamins <u>from within</u>. *The Journal of Nutrition* in 1999 noted that pantothenic acid is synthesized by intestinal microflora. The European Cancer Prevention Organization wrote, in a 1997 issue of the *European Journal of Cancer Prevention,* that:

> There is good evidence that the gut bacterial flora are a significant source of a range of vitamins to the human. In this paper evidence is presented that **gut bacteria are a significant source of a range of vitamins, particularly those of the B group and Vitamin K**.

From the journal *Gastroenterology*, 1996, Spanish researchers concluded that not only do the gut microflora synthesize folate, the "human host absorbs and uses some of these folates." From the journal *Nature*, 1980, researchers determined "the human small intestine also often harbours a considerable microflora.... We now show that at least two groups of organisms in the small bowel, *Pseudomonas* and *Klebsiella sp.*, may synthesize significant amounts of the vitamin," referring specifically to **Vitamin B-12**.

In a small way, so small that it's microscopic, the "Life Bridge" allies bring to life the inorganic compounds indispensable for human life. We've spoken here of "inside" and "outside" actions of microflora, but that is only meaningful from our human vantage point. From the perspective of the microflora—the view from the Bridge—there is no "inside" or "outside," there is only inorganic matter to culture and imbue with the wisdom of life. That is their gift to us. These timeless friends of animal life existed before us, but we could not exist without them.

A final note on B vitamins. We now understand they:
- are living vitamins born of the probiotic process;
- are more biologically effective or active in their living form; and
- arise from the beneficial actions of both *Saccharomyces cerevisiae* and *lactobacilli*.

This leads to some simple recommendations for B vitamin supplementation. First, it makes sense to have the Life Bridge allies working "within," so we feel that any vitamin supplement program starts with a probiotic source. That should include traditional whole foods that contain *live* active probiotic cultures, such as quality yogurts (milk, soy, almond, pine nut, and others), tempeh, miso, natto, beer, wine, kefir, fresh sauerkraut and kimchee. In addition, some foods are known to stimulate the growth of healthy "Life Bridge" allies, such as fresh fruit and vegetable fiber and foods containing whey. Certain spices, like cumin, chicory and ginger, are also highly effective in promoting probiotic colonization. There are also quality probiotic supplements available from a number of companies, and all of these, together, constitute an intelligent strategy for creating B and other vitamins "from within."

Other foods are bursting with natural, probiotic B vitamins, and we recommend them as well. Brewer's yeast from a reputable company like Lewis Labs is a natural starting place. We have recently come across a most interesting product that is "honey with a difference." This fascinating honey, from Israel, is made by bees fed nectar comprising honey and concentrates of Brewer's yeast and beer. The resulting "enriched" honey is apparently an excellent source of the B-complex vitamins, and we will be looking for this product should it come to the United States. There are also vitamin supplements that deliver all of the B vitamins in a probiotic form. When you consume a probiotic form of the B vitamins, you of course obtain the benefits of natural, living nutrients. Moreover, the co-factors created during the culturing process (SOD, phospholipids, beta-glucans, etc.) provide significant additional benefits. Finally, when the "Life Bridge" allies create the B vitamins, they do so in a manner to promote their own health. Such natural vitamin production is necessarily in balance with other cell enzymes, coenzymes, and compounds, and that gives comfort that the vitamin is in a biologically safe and reasonable form.

And finally, we end our Victory Lap, greeted by a tall glass of Dopplebock....

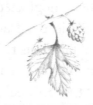

CHAPTER SIX

Nutrition: "To Us" or "With Us"

The role of microorganisms in the soil and their importance as contributors to and mediators of plant nutrition is not adequately recognized or fostered by most current methods of agriculture. Consequently, minerals and trace elements may become increasingly locked in that are unavailable to the plant that has access to them only in soluble form. Microorganisms are capable of dissolving and/or chelating these elements, thereby increasing their availability to plants.... Organic matter provides nutrition to soil microorganisms and provides medium for chelation... **A case can thus be made that our food plants are receiving a refined diet, lacking in micronutrients, just as our own diets have become refined**.
—*Nutritional Biochemistry*

We began this book with a recognition that nutritional supplementation has an indispensable role in promoting health and protecting us against many disease conditions. Perhaps, in some Golden Age of Agriculture when our water and air were pure and our plants and animals were vigorous and varied, humans could get all the nutrients they needed from an array of fresh, locally grown organic and cultured food. Sadly, that is not a reality for life in the early 21st Century. As the quotation starting this chapter illustrates, we have neglected our soil, failing to recognize that if the soil is dead and filled only with chemical isolates, critical nutrients remain locked in place and unavailable to our plants. It takes "living" soil, teeming with beneficial "Life Bridge" allies, to make those nutrients a living sustenance for the plants.

As Voltaire said at the end of *Candide*, "Well said, but we must go now and cultivate the garden." But what garden? Is it a grim conventional garden, where the soil is dead and all the nourishment comes from chemical fertilizers? Or is it an organic garden, where the soil is sweet smelling and alive with friendly "Life Bridge" allies that bind nutrients to the roots? Shall we garden with refined and isolated nitrogen and potassium, or use lower potencies of composted plants and manures? Is it a garden where we dump mega-potencies of nutrients into the soil, and the soil is just a holding pot for what we tell the plants they need? Or is it a garden where we replenish the humus and work with the soil, allowing the living soil to nourish the plants on their terms? That is the clear division facing us as gardeners.

And in our lives. We either see nutrition as something that happens to us, or that happens with us. The use of conventional USP-type supplements is the decision to have the chemicals dictate to us what we need, just like a drug or a chemical fertilizer. The use of food nourishment, such as with cultured nutrients, is the decision to have the living nutrients work with us. With probiotic nutrients, nutrition is "host mediated," relying on the innate wisdom of the body as it interacts with the healing genius of whole food.

We have presented the science, and we feel the medical evidence is compelling in favor of probiotic nutrients. Frankly, we don't even think it's a close call. But when all the science dust has settled, when the hurly-burly of the debate is done, aren't we left with our intuition as to what is right for us?

"Well said, but we must go now and cultivate the garden."

APPENDIX A

FERMENTED FOODS WORLDWIDE

Product name	Area of production	Substrate involved	Microorganisms	Characteristics
Coffee	Africa, Asia, Indonesia, and Latin America (Particularly Brazil, Columbia, Mexico, and Cote d'Ivoire)	Coffee beans (*Coffea arabica and Coffea canephora*)	*Leuconostoc mesenteroides, L. plantarum, L. brevis, Streptococcus faecalis, Aerobacter sp., Escherichia sp., Bacillus sp., Saccharomyces marscianus, S. bayanus, Flavobacterium sp., Erwinia dissolvens, Fusarium sp., Aspergillus sp., Penicillium.*	Beverage
Vanilla	Madagascar, Indonesia, and various Pacific Islands	Orchids of genus *Vanilla* usually *V. planifolia* or *V. fragrans*	*	Seasoning
Red Grape Wine	World Wide	Grapes (*Vitis vinifera*)	*S. cerevisiae*	Alcoholic beverage
White Grape Wine	World Wide	Grapes (*Vitis vinifera*)	*S. cerevisiae*	Alcoholic beverage
Cocoa Powder	Africa, Asia, Indonesia, Latin America (particularly Cote d'Ivoire, Ghana, and Brazil)	Cocoa plant (*Theobroma cacao*)	*S. cerevisiae, Candida krusei, Kloeckra apiculata, Pichia fermentans, Hansenula anomola, Schizo-saccharomyces pombe*	Powder

* Unknown

FERMENTED FOODS WORLDWIDE

Product name	Area of production	Substrate involved	Microorganisms	Characteristics
Chocolate	World Wide	Cocoa plant (Theobroma cacao)	S. cerevisiae, Candida krusei, Kloeckra apiculata, Pichia fermentans, Hansenula anomola, Schizo-saccharomyces pombe	Solid
Kefir	World Wide	Milk	Lactobacillus spp.	Liquid
Yogurt	World Wide	Milk	Lactobacillus acidophilus, L. bulgaricus, S. thermophillus	
Calpis	Japan	Milk	L. helviticus, S. cerevisiae	Beverage
Yakult	Japan	Milk	L. Shirota	Beverage
Fermented Soy Milk	World Wide	Soy milk	Bifidobacterium breve	Liquid
Sourdough	Worldwide	Almost any cereal grain	S. cerevisiae, Candida pelliculosa, Leuconostoc spp., L breve, L. curvatus, L. lactis ssp. Lactis, Lactococcus lactis ssp. lactis, Enterococcus casseliflavus, E. durans, E. faecium, Streptococcus constellantus, S. equinus, L.sanfranciscensis, L. reuteri, L. pontis	Dough
Kimchee	Korea	Vegetable	Lactobacillus kimchii sp. nov.	Side dish

* Unknown

FERMENTED FOODS WORLDWIDE

Product name	Area of production	Substrate involved	Microorganisms	Characteristics
Natto	Japan	Soybean	*Bacillus natto*	Seasoning
Miso	Japan	Soybean	*Aspergillus oryzae*	
Sofu or furu	China	Soybean	*Actinomucor spp., Mucor spp., and Rhizopus spp.*	Side dish
Tempeh	Indonesia	Soybean	*Rhizopus spp.*	Seasoning
Sauerkraut	Europe, US	Cabbage	*L. curvatus, L. sake*	Side dish
Mead	Worldwide	Honey, fruit	*S. cerevisiae*	Alcoholic beverage
Beer	Worldwide	Wheat, hops	*Lactobacillus spp., and yeasts*	Alcoholic beverage
Tempoyak	Malaysia	Durain fruit (*Durio zibethinus*)	*L. plantarum, L. brevis, Leuconstoc mesenteroides, L. mali, L. fermentum, and unidentified Lactobacillus spp*	Condiment
Dawadawa	Africa	African locust bean	*Bacillus subtilis*	Beverage
Saumbala	Africa	African locust bean	*Bacillus subtilis*	Beverage
Kinema	Africa	Soybean	*Bacillus subtilis*	Beverage
Boza	Bulgaria	Cereals	*	Beverage
Doli Ki Roti	India	Wheat, chick peas	*	Dough

*Unknown

FERMENTED FOODS WORLDWIDE

Product name	Area of production	Substrate involved	Microorganisms	Characteristics
Cheeses-blue veined	Europe, US	Milk	*Debaryomyces hansenii, Saccharomyces spp. especially S. cerevisiae*	Solid
Artisanal cheeses	Europe	Raw milks-goat, sheep, cow, and/or buffalo	*S. cerevisiae, Kluyveromyces marxianus, K. lactis, Candida kefir, Debaryomyces hansenii, C. famata, C. colliculosa, C. Catenulata, Trichosporon cutaneum, Yarrowia lipolytica*	Solid
Idli	South India Sri Lanka	Rice grits and black gram powder	*L. mesenteroides S. fecalis, T. candida, T. pullulans*	Steamed cake
Dosa	India	Rice flour and black gram powder	*L. mesenteroides, S. faecalis, T. candida, T. pullulans*	Griddled pancake
Nazerushi	Japan	Salt water fish, cooked millet, and salt	*L. mesenteroides, L. plantarum*	Side dish
Ogi	Nigeria, Benin	Maize, sorghum, or millet	*Lactobacillus sp and yeasts*	Soft or stiff gel
Bogobe Koko and Kenkey	Botswana and Ghana	Sorghum and maize, sorghum, or millet	*Unknown Lactobacillus sp and yeasts*	Porridge Dough

*Unknown

FERMENTED FOODS WORLDWIDE

Product name	Area of production	Substrate involved	Microorganisms *L. fermentum, L. cellobiosis, L. brevis, Candida krusei, and S. cervisiae*	Characteristics
Mawe	Dahomey	Maize		Dough
Injera	Ethiopia	Sorghum	*	Paste
Sendecho	Mexico	Germinated maize and red chili	*	Alcoholic beverage
Sora	Peru	Germinated and cooked maize	*	Alcoholic beverage
Tepache	Mexico	Maize grains and brown sugar	*	Alcoholic beverage
Tesguino	Mexico	Germinated, ground, and cooked maize with fragments of plant leaves	*	Alcoholic beverage
Tocos	Peru	Maize	*	Dessert
Zarzaparrilla bark wine	Mexico	Maize and zarzaparrilla bark	*	Alcoholic beverage

*Unknown

FERMENTED FOODS WORLDWIDE

Product name	Area of production	Substrate involved	Microorganisms	Characteristics
Zambumbia	Mexico	Toasted barley	*	Alcoholic beverage
Dhokla	India	Rice and bengal gram	L. mesenteroides, S. faecalis, T. candida, T. Pullulans	Steamed cake
Jalebies	India, Nepal, and Pakistan	Wheat flour	S. bayanus	Pretzel-like confection
Mantou	China	Wheat flour	Saccharomyces spp.	Steamed cake
Kichudok	Korea	Rice, takju	Saccharomyces spp.	Steamed cake
Puto	Philippines	Rice, sugar	L. mesenteroides, S. faecalis yeast	Steamed cake
Brem	Indonesia	Glutinous rice	*	Cake
Mungbean starch	China, Thailand, Korea, and Japan	Mungbean starch	L. mesenteroides, L. casei, L. cellobiosus, L. fermenti	Noodle
Khanomjeen	Thailand	Rice	Lactobacillus sp., Streptococcus sp.	Noodle
Me	Vietnam	Rice	Lactic acid bacteria	Sour food ingredient

*Unknown

FERMENTED FOODS WORLDWIDE

Product name	Area of production	Substrate involved	Microorganisms	Characteristics
Sikhae	Korea	Salt water fish, cooked millet, and salt	L. mesenteroides, L. plantarum	Side dish
Burong-isda	Philippines	Fresh water fish, rice, and salt	L. brevis, Streptococcus sp.	Side dish
Pla-ra and Pla-chom	Thailand	Fresh water fish, salt, and roasted rice	Pediococcus sp.	Side dish
Balao-balao	Philippines	Shrimp, rice, and salt	L. mesenteroides, P. cerevisiae	Side dish
Kungchao	Thailand	Fresh water fish and sweet rice	P. cerevisiae	Side dish
Nham	Thailand	Pork meat in banana leaves, salt ,rice, and garlic	P. cerevisiae, L. brevis , L. plantarum	Main dish
Toddy	Asia (particularly India and Sri Lanka)	Sap of Coconut Palm	small amount of toddy left in the pot	Alcoholic beverage
Pulque	Mexico	Various cacti	S. carbajali, L. plantarum, Leuconstoc sp.	Alcoholic beverage

*Unknown

FERMENTED FOODS WORLDWIDE

Product name	Area of production	Substrate involved	Microorganisms	Characteristics
Nipa Palm vinegar	East Asia (particularly Papua New Guinea)	Nipa Palm	*	Seasoning
Tabasco	Mexico and Guatemala	Chili pods	*	Seasoning
Sai-krok-prieo	Thailand	Pork, rice, garlic, salt	*L. plantarum, L. salivarius, P. Pentosaccus*	Sausage
Nem-chua	Vietnam	Pork, salt, cooked rice	*Pediococcus sp., Lactobacillus s?.*	Sausage
Banana Beer	Africa	Bananas, cereal flour	*S. cerevisiae*	Alcoholic beverage
Cashew wine	Asia and Latin America	Fruit of cashew tree	*S. cerevisiae*	Alcoholic beverage
Cachaca (aguardente)	Brazil	Sugar cane juice	*S. cerevisiae, Rhodoturula glutinis, Candida maltosa*	Alcoholic beverage
Tepache	Mexico	Maize, pineapple, apples, or oranges	*B. subtilis, B. graveolus, Torulopsis insconspicna, S. cerevisiae, Candida queretana*	Beverage

*Unknown

109

FERMENTED FOODS WORLDWIDE

Product name	Area of production	Substrate involved	Microorganisms	Characteristics
Colonche	Mexico	Fruits of prickly pear cactus	*	Beverage
Date wine	Sudan and North Africa	Dates	*	Alcoholic beverage
Jack-fruit wine	India	Jack-fruit (*Artocarous heterophyllus*)	*inoculum from previous wine*	Alcoholic beverage
Palm wine	West Africa	Palm sap	*S. cerevisiae, Schizosaccharomyces pombe, L. plantarum, L. mesenteroides*	Alcoholic beverage
Mahewu (magou)	South Africa	Maize sorghum or millet	*L. delbruckii , L. bulgaricus*	Liquid
Uji	East Africa	Maize, sorghum, or millet and sorghum	*	Liquid
Kisra	Sudan	Sorghum	*	Dough
Enjara	Ethiopia	Sorghum	*Candida guilliermondii yeasts*	Dough

*Unknown

FERMENTED FOODS WORLDWIDE

Product name	Area of production	Substrate involved	Microorganisms	Characteristics
Kishk	Egypt and most Arab countries	Parboiled milk and wheat	*L. plantarum, L. brevis, L. casei, Bacillus subtilis, yeasts*	Paste
Gari	Northern Guinea region of Nigeria, Benin, andGhana	Cassava	*	Farinaceous
Burukutu	Northern Guinea region of Nigeria, Benin, and Ghana	Sorghum	*S. cerevisae, S. chavelieri, Leuconostoc mesetercides*	Alcoholic beverage
PitoKaffir beer	Nigeria, Ghana	Maize, sorghum, or maize and sorghum	*Geotrichum candidum, Lactobacillus sp>, Candida sp.*	Alcoholic beverage
Busaa (maize beer)	Nigeria (Bendel), Ghana	Kaffir corn (or maize)	*Lactobacillus spp>, yeasts*	Alcoholic beverage
Malawa beer	South Africa	Maize	*Yeasts, Lactobacillus spp.*	Alcoholic beverage
Zambian opaquemaize beer	East Africa	Maize	*Candida krusei*	Alcoholic beverage

*Unknown

111

FERMENTED FOODS WORLDWIDE

Product name	Area of production	Substrate involved	Microorganisms	Characteristics
Merissa	Uganda	Maize	*Yeasts*	Alcoholic beverage
Seketeh	Zambia	Sorghum	*Lactic acid bacteria, acetic acid bacteria*	Alcoholic beverage
Bouza	Egypt	Wheat	*	Alcoholic beverage
Talla	Nigeria (south)	Maize	*	Alcoholic beverage
Kanu-Zaki	Nigeria	Millet	*Lactic acid bacteria, yeasts*	Beverage
Shaosinghjiu	China	Rice	*S. cerevisiae*	Alcoholic beverage
Chongju	Korea	Rice	*S. cerevisiae*	Alcoholic beverage
Sale	Japan	Rice	*S. sake*	Alcoholic beverage
Takju	Korea	Rice, wheat	*Lactic acid bacteria, S. cerevisiae*	Alcoholic beverage
Tapuy	Philippines	Rice, glutinous rice	*Saccharomyces Mucor, Aspergillus Leuconostoc, L.Plantarum ,Rhizopus*	Alcoholic beverage and paste
Brembali	Indonesia	Glutinous rice	*Mucor indicus, Candida*	Alcoholic beverage

*Unknown

112

FERMENTED FOODS WORLDWIDE

Product name	Area of production	Substrate involved	Microorganisms	Characteristics
Jaanr	India	Finger millet	*Hansenula Himalaya anomala, Mucor rouxianus*	Sweet-sour alcoholic paste; mix with water
Khaomak	Thailand	Glutinous rice	*Rhizopus, Mucor alcoholic, Saccharomyces, Hansenula*	Semisolid, sweet
Tapai pulut	Malaysia	Glutinous rice	*Chlamydomucor, Endomycopsis alcoholic, Hansenula*	Semisolid, sweet
Tape-ketan	Indonesia	Glutinous rice and rice	*A. rouxii, E. burtonii, E. fibuliger*	Sweet-sour alcoholic paste
Lao-chao	China	Rice	*Rhizopus, A. rouxii*	Paste
Bhattejaanr	India	Glutinous rice	*Hansenula anomala, Mucor rouxianus*	Sweet-sour alcoholic paste
Mirin	Japan	Rice, alcohol	*A. oryzae, A. usamii*	Alcoholic liquid seasoning
Abati	Paraguay, Argentina	Maize	*	Alcoholic beverage

*Unknown

113

FERMENTED FOODS WORLDWIDE

Product name	Area of production	Substrate involved	Microorganisms	Characteristics
Fuba	Brazil	Germinated Maize	*	Granular
Jaminbang	Brazil	Maize	*	Dough
Napu	Peru	Germinated and ground Maize	*	Beverage
Ostoche	Mexico	Maize juice, pulque, or brown sugar	*	Alcoholic beverage
Pozol	Mexico	Maize	*	Beverage
Quebranta huesos	Mexico	Maize juice, toasted maize, and piru fruits	*	Alcoholic beverage
Kivunde	China, Tanzania, Uganda, Zaire	Cassava	L. plantarum	Dough
Tarhana	Turkey	Wheat flour, yogurt, yeast, cooked tomatoes, onions, and green peppers, salt, mint, and paprika	lactic acid bacteria, yeast	Soup

*Unknown

114

FERMENTED FOODS WORLDWIDE

Product name	Area of production	Substrate involved	Microorganisms	Characteristics
Surstromming	Sweden	Herring	*Haloanaerobium praevalens* or *Haloanaerobium alcaliphilum*	Side dish
Mukumbi	Zimbabwe	*Sclerocarya birrea ssp. caffra* tree fruit	*	Alcoholic beverage
Wara	Nigeria	Skimmed cow's milk	*Lactococcus lactis, Enterococcus faecium*	Solid
Kpaye	Africa	*Prosopis africana* seeds	*Bacillus subtilis, B. lichenformis, B. pumilus*	Condiment
Sparish green olives	Europe, US	Green olives	*Lactobacillus plantarum ssp.*	Condiment
Raib	Morocco	Milk	*Lactococcus lactis ssp., Enteroccus Faecium ssp., E. faecalis ssp.*	Beverage

*Unknown

115

APPENDIX B

Partial List of Beneficial Compounds Created by Probiotics

Adenosyl-methionine
Antimicrobial peptides
ATP
Bacteriocins (numerous)
Beta Glucans
Biosurfacants
Biocytin
Biotin
Casein Phosphatase
Coenzyme A
Conjugated Linoleic Acid (CLA)
Cysteine
Diacetyl
FAD
Folic Acid
Glutathione
GTF Chromium
Hydrogen Peroxide
Immune-enhancing Peptides
Lactic Acid
Lipoic Acid
Lysozyme
NAD
NADP
Pantetheine
Peptidoglycans
Phosphaditylcholine
Phosphaditylethanolamine
Phosphaditylinositol
Phosphaditylserine
Pyridoxal
Pyridoxamine
Pyridoxamine Phosphate
Reuterin
Teichoic Acid
Unidentified ACE Inhibitors
Unidentified Antimutagens
Vitamin B1 (thiamin)
Vitamin B2 (riboflavin)
Vitamin B3 (nicotinic acid)
Vitamin B5 (pantothenic acid)
Vitamin B12
Vitamin B13 (orotic acid)
Vitamin D
Vitamin F
Volatile Fatty Acids-Acetic, Propionic, and Butyric
6-hydroxydaidzein
8-hydroxydaidzein
8-hydroxygenistein

Stage 1A: Preparation for Culturing

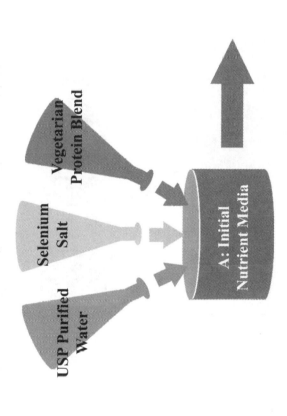

A: In one tank, U.S.P. purified water, Selenium salt (or other mineral salts or vitamins) and a vegetarian protein blend are mixed together.

Stage 1B: Preparation for Culturing

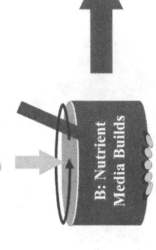

Natural
Bioflavonoids
Added

B: Nutrient
Media Builds

B: The solution is gently warmed and stirred for many hours, then natural bioflavonoids are added to increase stability.

Stage 1C: Preparation for Culturing

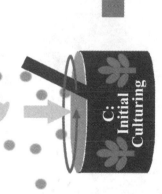

Non-GMO Nutritional Yeast and Plant Carbohydrates

C: Initial Culturing

C: Simultaneously in a separate tank, natural, non-GMO nutritional yeast solution is mixed with natural plant carbohydrates.

Stage 2: Advanced Culturing Process

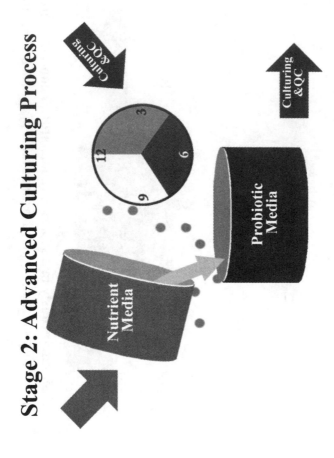

The U.S.P. Nutrient Media is added into the Active Yeast Solution to culture for 4 to 8 hours.

Stage 3: Soy Culture Phase

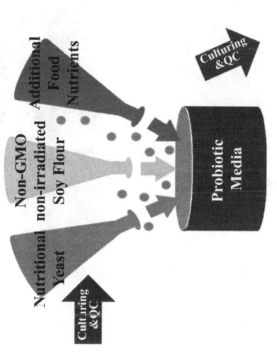

We now add nutritional yeast, non-GMO, non-irradiated soy flour and additional food nutrients (e.g. carrots, oranges, etc.) specific to the vitamin or mineral formulation.

Stage 4: Culturing Deceleration

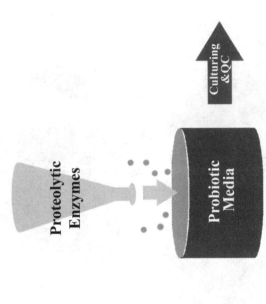

Proteolytic Enzymes are now added to break the
nutritional yeast cell wall and slow the culturing process.

Stage 5: Lactobacilli Culturing

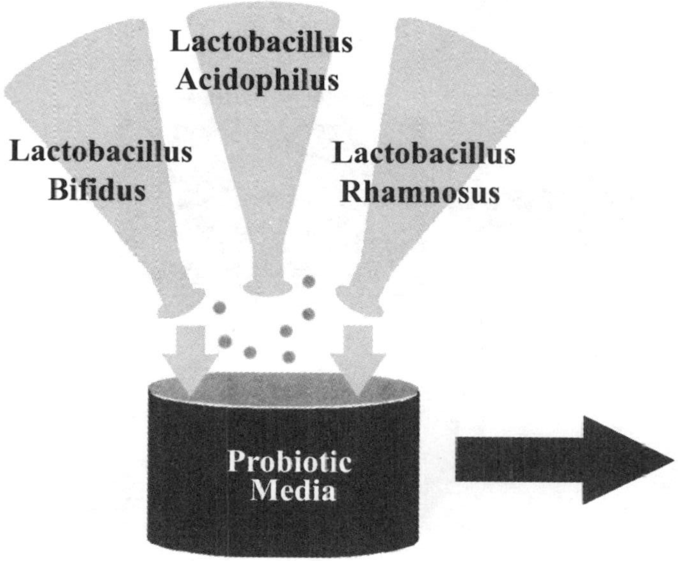

Lactobacillus Acidophilus

Lactobacillus Rhamnosus

Lactobacillus Bifidus

Probiotic Media

Three strains of Lactobacilli culture the nutrients to additionally activate.

Stage 6: Low-heat Culturing Deactivation Phase

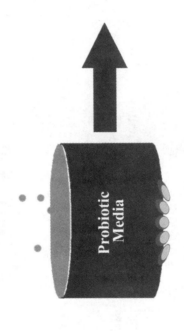

Probiotic Media

Low heat is applied to completely deactivate the live culturing process.

Stage 7: Proprietary Spray Drying

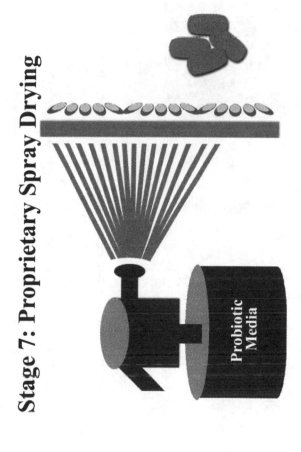

Probiotic Nutrients undergo
proprietary spray drying to preserve all active ingredients—
easy to digest; with maximum activity, bioavailability and stability.

Stage 8: Analysis of Biological Activity

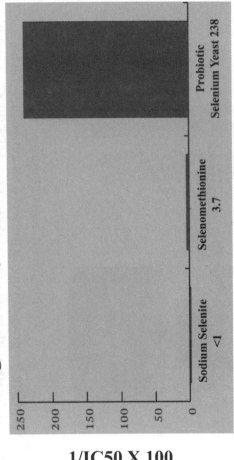

Probiotic Nutrients undergo HPLC and other laboratory analyses to determine stability and bioactivity. Our tests show that probiotic Selenium is a vastly superior antioxidant. In this analysis, "Sodium selenite exhibited no antioxidant activity and the Selenium Yeast was 64 X better as an antioxidant than selenomethionine. Also the Selenium Yeast was better than the vitamin C, E and beta carotene."

Analysis performed at the University of Scranton by Dr. Joe A. Vinson, PhD, one of the world's leading antioxidant researchers.

APPENDIX D

Sample Health Benefits of Select Lactobacilli Strains

LACTOBACILLUS ACIDOPHILUS

Reduces mutagenicity in colon and risk of cancer
J Dairy Sci 1996 May;79(5):745-9 Effect of administration of milk fermented with Lactobacillus acidophilus LA-2 on fecal mutagenicity and microflora in the human intestine. Hosoda M, Hashimoto H, He F, Morita H, Hosono A. Technical Research Laboratory, Takanashi Milk Products Co., Ltd, Yokohama, Japan. PMID: 8792276

Eur J Cancer Prev 1992 Aug;1(5):341-53 Lactobacilli, anticarcinogenic activities and human intestinal microflora. Lidbeck A, Nord CE, Gustafsson JA, Rafter J. Department of Microbiology, Huddinge University Hospital, Karolinska Institute, Sweden. PMID: 1463986

J Dairy Sci 1994 Nov;77(11):3287-95 Antimutagenicity of fermented milk. Nadathur SR, Gould SJ, Bakalinsky AT. Department of Food Science and Technology, Oregon State University, Corvallis 97331. PMID: 7814704

Eur J Cancer Prev 1992 Aug;1(5):341-53 Lactobacilli, anticarcinogenic activities and human intestinal microflora. Lidbeck A, Nord CE, Gustafsson JA, Rafter J. Department of Microbiology, Huddinge University Hospital, Karolinska Institute, Sweden. PMID: 1463986

Supernatant shows anti-tumor effects and breast cancer cell line.
Nutr Cancer 1997;28(1):93-9 Antiproliferative effect of fermented milk on the growth of a human breast cancer cell line. Biffi A, Coradini D, Larsen R, Riva L, Di Fronzo G. Istituto Nazionale per lo Studio e la Cura dei Tumori, Milan, Italy.PMID: 9200156

Counters vaginal candidal colonization and infection
Arzneimittelforschung 1996 Jan;46(1):68-73 Therapy of bacterial vaginosis using exogenously-applied Lactobacilli acidophili and a low dose of estriol: a placebo-controlled multicentric clinical trial. Parent D, Bossens M, Bayot D, Kirkpatrick C, Graf F, Wilkinson FE, Kaiser RR. Hopital Universitaire Erasme, Brussels, Belgium. PMID: 8821521

Sex Transm Dis 1992 May-Jun;19(3):146-8 Treatment of bacterial vaginosis with lactobacilli. Hallen A, Jarstrand C, Pahlson C. Department of Dermatology and Venereology, University Hospital, Uppsala, Sweden. PMID: 1523530

JAMA 1996 Mar 20;275(11):870-6 JAMA. 1996 Jul 3;276(1):29-30 Biotherapeutic agents. A neglected modality for the treatment and prevention of selected intestinal and vaginal infections. Elmer GW, Surawicz CM, McFarland LV. Department of Medicinal Chemistry, School of Pharmacy, University of Washington, Seattle 98195, USA. PMID: 8596226

Microbios 1994;80(323):125-33 Inhibition of Candida albicans by Lactobacillus acidophilus: evidence for the involvement of a peroxidase system. Fitzsimmons N, Berry DR. Microbiology Laboratory, Crosshouse Hospital, Kilmarnock, Scotland.PMID: 7898374

Ann Intern Med 1992 Mar 1;116(5):353-7 Comment in: Ann Intern Med. 1992 Aug 15;117(4):345-6 Ann Intern Med. 1992 Mar 1;116(5):419-20 Ingestion of yogurt containing Lactobacillus acidophilus as prophylaxis for candidal vaginitis. Hilton E, Isenberg HD, Alperstein P, France K, Borenstein MT. Division of Infectious Diseases, Long Island Jewish Medical Center, New Hyde Park, NY 11042.PMID: 1736766

Microbios 1990;62(250):37-46 Evidence for the involvement of thiocyanate in the inhibition of Candida albicans by Lactobacillus acidophilus. Jack M, Wood BJ, Berry DR. Department of Bioscience and Biotechnology, University of Strathclyde, Glasgow, Scotland, Great Britain.PMID: 2110612

J Dairy Sci 1980 May;63(5):830-2 Inhibition of Candida albicans by Lactobacillus acidophilus. Collins EB, Hardt P.PMID: 6771309

Microbios 1994;80(323):125-33 Inhibition of Candida albicans by Lactobacillus acidophilus: evidence for the involvement of a peroxidase system. Fitzsimmons N, Berry DR. Microbiology Laboratory, Crosshouse Hospital, Kilmarnock, Scotland.PMID: 7898374

Ann Intern Med 1992 Mar 1;116(5):353-7 Comment in: Ann Intern Med. 1992 Aug 15;117(4):345-6 Ann Intern Med. 1992 Mar 1;116(5):419-20 Ingestion of yogurt containing Lactobacillus acidophilus as prophylaxis for candidal vaginitis. Hilton E, Isenberg HD, Alperstein P, France K, Borenstein MT. Division of Infectious Diseases, Long Island Jewish Medical Center, New Hyde Park, NY 11042. PMID: 1736766

Infect Dis Obstet Gynecol 2001;9(1):33-9 Antimicrobial protein produced by vaginal Lactobacillus acidophilus that inhibits Gardnerella vaginalis. Aroutcheva AA, Simoes JA, Faro S. Department of Obstetrics and Gynecology, Rush-Presbyterian-St. Luke's Medical Center, Chicago, IL 60612, USA. PMID: 11368257

J Med Microbiol 2000 Jun;49(6):543-52 Characterisation and selection of a Lactobacillus species to re-colonise the vagina of women with recurrent bacterial vaginosis. McLean NW, Rosenstein IJ. Imperial College of Science, Technology and Medicine, Department of GenitoUrinary Medicine, London. PMID: 10847208

May play a role in prevention of HIV transmission.
J Exp Med 1991 Jul 1;174(1):289-92 Viricidal effect of Lactobacillus acidophilus on human immunodeficiency virus type 1: possible role in heterosexual transmission. Klebanoff SJ, Coombs RW. Department of Medicine, University of Washington, Seattle 98195.PMID: 1647436

Potentiates immune functioning
Immunology 1988 Jan;63(1):17-23 Systemic augmentation of the immune response in mice by feeding fermented milks with Lactobacillus casei and Lactobacillus acidophilus. Perdigon G, de Macias ME, Alvarez S, Oliver G, de Ruiz Holgado AP. Centro de Referencia para Lactobacilos (CERELA), Chacabuco, Tucuman, Argentina.PMID: 3123370

Aids in the modulation or reduction of cholesterol
J Dairy Sci 1990 Apr;73(4):905-11 Factors to consider when selecting a culture of Lactobacillus acidophilus as a dietary adjunct to produce a hypocholesterolemic effect in humans. Gilliland SE, Walker DK. Animal Science Department, Oklahoma State University, Stillwater 74078-0425. PMID: 2111831

Appl Environ Microbiol 1985 Feb;49(2):377-81 Assimilation of cholesterol by Lactobacillus acidophilus. Gilliland SE, Nelson CR, Maxwell C. PMID: 3920964

128

Folia Microbiol (Praha) 2000;45(3):263-8 Verification of hypocholesterolemic effect of fermented milk on human subjects with different cholesterol levels. Ashar MN, Prajapati JB. Dairy Microbiology Department, SMC College of Dairy Science, Gujarat Agricultural University, Anand 388 110, India. PMID: 11271813

J Am Coll Nutr 1999 Feb;18(1):43-50 Effect of fermented milk (yogurt) containing Lactobacillus acidophilus L1 on serum cholesterol in hypercholesterolemic humans. Anderson JW, Gilliland SE. Metabolic Research Group, VA Medical Center, University of Kentucky, Lexington 40511, USA. PMID: 10067658

Eur J Clin Nutr 1998 Jun;52(6):436-40 Effects of a milk product, fermented by Lactobacillus acidophilus and with fructo-oligosaccharides added, on blood lipids in male volunteers. Schaafsma G, Meuling WJ, van Dokkum W, Bouley C. TNO Nutrition and Food Research Institute, Zeist, The Netherlands. PMID: 9683397

Supernatant and live cells show long-term suppresive effect on H. Pylori and other pathological species

J Clin Microbiol 1989 Oct;27(10):2328-30 Lactobacillus acidophilus inhibits growth of Campylobacter pylori in vitro. Bhatia SJ, Kochar N, Abraham P, Nair NG, Mehta AP. Department of Gastroenterology, King Edward Memorial Hospital, Bombay, India.PMID: 2511224

Curr Microbiol 2001 Jan;42(1):39-44 Lactobacillus acidophilus autolysins inhibit Helicobacter pylori in vitro. Lorca GL, Wadstrom T, Valdez GF, Ljungh A. Centro de Referencia para Lactobacilos (CERELA), Chacabuco 145, 4000 Tucuman, Argentina. PMID: 11116395

Med Dosw Mikrobiol 1999;51(1-2):47-57 [The range of antagonistic effects of Lactobacillus bacterial strains on etiologic agents of bacterial vaginosis] Strus M, Malinowska M. Zaklad Bakteriologii Instytutu Mikrobiologii Collegium Medicum Uniwersytetu Jagiellonskiego w Krakowie. PMID: 10865430

Digestion 1999;60(3):203-9 Effect of whey-based culture supernatant of Lactobacillus acidophilus (johnsonii) La1 on Helicobacter pylori infection in humans. Michetti P, Dorta G, Wiesel PH, Brassart D, Verdu E, Herranz M, Felley C, Porta N, Rouvet M, Blum AL, Corthesy-Theulaz I. Division of Gastroenterology, Department of Medicine, University Hospital, Lausanne, Switzerland. pmichett@bidmc.harvard.edu PMID: 10343133

Appl Environ Microbiol 1997 Jul;63(7):2747-53 The human Lactobacillus acidophilus strain LA1 secretes a nonbacteriocin antibacterial substance(s) active in vitro and in vivo. Bernet-Camard MF, Lievin V, Brassart D, Neeser JR, Servin AL, Hudault S. CJF 94.07 INSERM, UFR de Pharmacie, Universite Paris XI, F-92296 Chatenay-Malabry, France. PMID: 9212421

Antimicrob Agents Chemother 1997 May;41(5):1046-52 Antibacterial effect of the adhering human Lactobacillus acidophilus strain LB. Coconnier MH, Lievin V, Bernet-Camard MF, Hudault S, Servin AL. CJF 94.07 INSERM, UFR de Pharmacie Paris XI, Chatenay-Malabry, France. PMID: 9145867

Appl Environ Microbiol 1998 Nov;64(11):4573-80 Antagonistic activity against Helicobacter infection in vitro and in vivo by the human Lactobacillus acidophilus strain LB. Coconnier MH, Lievin V, Hemery E, Servin AL. Institut National de la Sante et de la Recherche Medicale, CJF 94. 07, UFR de Pharmacie, Universite Paris XI, F-92296 Chatenay-Malabry, France.PMID: 9797324

Med Pregl 1998 Jul-Aug;51(7-8):343-5 [Therapy of Helicobacter pylori infection using Lactobacillus acidophilus] Mrda Z, Zivanovic M, Rasic J, Gajin S, Somer L, Trbojevic S, Majoros J, Petrovic Z. Institut za interne bolesti, Medicinski Fakultet, Novi Sad. PMID: 9769669

Reduces lactose intolerance and dyspepsia after antibiotics

Vnitr Lek 1994 Feb;40(2):79-83 [Lactobacilli in the treatment of dyspepsia due to dysmicrobia of various causes] Kocian J. Interni katedra Institutu postgradualniho vzdelavani zdravotniku, Praha. PMID: 8140765

Counters maldigestion, malabsorption, radiation enterocolitis and negative digestive effects of antibiotics

Vnitr Lek 1994 Feb;40(2):79-83 [Lactobacilli in the treatment of dyspepsia due to dysmicrobia of various causes] Kocian J. Interni katedra Institutu postgradualniho vzdelavani zdravotniku, Praha. PMID: 8140765

Reduces acute symptoms of gastrointestinal toxicity from radiation therapy

Strahlenther Onkol 1998 Nov;174 Suppl 3:82-4 Radiation-induced gastrointestinal toxicity. Pathophysiology, approaches to treatment and prophylaxis. Classen J, Belka C, Paulsen F, Budach W, Hoffmann W, Bamberg M. Abteilung für Strahlentherapie der Universitat Tubingen. johannes.classen@uni-tuebingen.de PMID: 9830465

Helps prevent development of Klebsiella infection

Fiziol Zh 1993 Jul-Aug;39(4):62-8 [Protective effect of Lactobacillus acidophilus on development of infection, caused by Klebsiella pneumoniae] Kostiuk OP, Chernyshova LI, Slukvin II.PMID: 8243718

Heat stable factor produced by acidophilus inhibits E coli adhesion.

Ann Rech Vet 1992;23(4):361-70 Heat-killed Lactobacillus acidophilus inhibits adhesion of Escherichia coli B41 to HeLa cells. Fourniat J, Colomban C, Linxe C, Karam D. Faculte de Pharmacie, Laboratoire de Microbiologie, Chatenay-Malabry, France. PMID: 1476406

Inhibitory and bactericidal Against E. Coli

Int J Food Microbiol 2001 Aug 15;68(1-2):135-40 Inhibition of in vitro growth of Shiga toxin-producing Escherichia coli O157:H7 by probiotic Lactobacillus strains due to production of lactic acid. Ogawa M, Shimizu K, Nomoto K, Tanaka R, Hamabata T, Yamasaki S, Takeda T, Takeda Y. Yakult Central Institute for Microbiologial Research, Kunitachi, Tokyo, Japan. PMID: 11545213

Resists streptococcol tonsillitis

Lik Sprava 2000 Jan-Feb;(1):79-82 [The development of a treatment method for streptococcal tonsillitis in children] Marushko IV.PMID: 10878987

Prophylaxis and treatment of cholera

Zh Mikrobiol Epidemiol Immunobiol 2001 Mar-Apr;(2):68-71 [Experimental evaluation of efficacy of Lactobacilli in prophylaxis and treatment of cholera] Bardykh ID, Krylikov VD, Mazrukho BL, Ryzhko IV, Moskvitina EA, Tsuraeva RI, Vinokur NI, Drobotkovskaia NV. Research Institute for Plague Control, Rostov-on-Don, Russia. PMID: 11548265

Induces interferon
Microbiol Immunol 1992;36(3):311-5 Interferon induction in murine peritoneal macrophage by stimulation with Lactobacillus acidophilus. Kitazawa H, Matsumura K, Itoh T, Yamaguchi T. Laboratory of Animal Products Chemistry, Faculty of Agriculture, Tohoku University, Miyagi, Japan. PMID: 1603000

Non-viable acidophilus strain enhances immunoglobulin levels
Zh Mikrobiol Epidemiol Immunobiol 1992;(11-12):12-5 [The effect of Lactobacillus acidophilus "Solco" on the immunological indices of totally decontaminated mice under complete gnotobiological isolation] Smeianov VV, Mal'tseva NN, Bossart W, Korshunov VM.PMID: 1301651

Produces immunosupportive and protective bacteriocins
Antimicrob Agents Chemother 1984 Sep;26(3):328-34 Purification and characterization of the Lactobacillus acidophilus bacteriocin lactacin B. Barefoot SF, Klaenhammer TR.PMID: 6439113

Appl Environ Microbiol 1983 Jun;45(6):1808-15 Detection and activity of lactacin B, a bacteriocin produced by Lactobacillus acidophilus. Barefoot SF, Klaenhammer TR.PMID: 6410990

Antibiotiki 1981 Nov;26(11):843-7 [Bacteriocin properties of Lactobacillus acidophilus] Filippov VA.PMID: 6798923

Extracts demonstrate significant antioxidant and SOD activity.
Chem Pharm Bull (Tokyo) 1989 Nov;37(11):3026-8 Superoxide dismutase activity in some strains of lactobacilli: induction by manganese. Gonzalez SN, Apella MC, Romero N, Pesce de Ruiz Holgado AA, Oliver G.PMID: 2632048

Dig Dis Sci 2000 Aug;45(8):1617-22 Antioxidative effect of intestinal bacteria Bifidobacterium longum ATCC 15708 and Lactobacillus acidophilus ATCC 4356. Lin MY, Chang FJ. Department of Food Science, National Chung Hsing University, Taichung, Taiwan.PMID: 11007114

J Agric Food Chem 1999 Apr;47(4):1460-6 Antioxidative ability of lactic acid bacteria. Lin MY, Yen CL. Department of Food Science, National Chung Hsing University, Taiwan. PMID: 10563999

Production of wide range of health supportive compounds
Crit Rev Microbiol 1995;21(3):175-214 Anticarcinogenic, hypocholesterolemic, and antagonistic activities of Lactobacillus acidophilus. Mital BK, Garg SK. Department of Food Science and Technology, G. B. Pant University of Agriculture and Technology, Nainital, India.PMID: 8845062

Increases iron bioavailability
J Nutr Sci Vitaminol (Tokyo) 1994 Dec;40(6):613-6 Effect of Lactobacillus acidophilus on iron bioavailability in rats. Oda T, Kado-oka Y, Hashiba H. Technical Research Institute, Snow Brand Milk Products Co. Ltd., Kawagoe, Japan.PMID: 7751979

LACTOBACILLUS BIFIDUS

Improves lactose digestion
Am J Clin Nutr 1991 Dec;54(6):1041-6 Strains and species of lactic acid bacteria in fermented milks (yogurts): effect on in vivo lactose digestion. Martini MC, Lerebours EC, Lin WJ, Harlander SK, Berrada NM, Antoine JM, Savaiano DA. Department of Food Science and Nutrition, University of Minnesota, St Paul 55108. PMID: 1957819

Aids digestion in immunologically compromised individuals
Gematol Transfuziol 1989 Jan;34(1):11-4 [Bacteriotherapy of intestinal dysbacteriosis in patients with acute leukemia] [Article in Russian] Tolkacheva TV, Abakumov EM, Golosova TV, Volodina NI.PMID: 2721896

Supresses potentially toxic bacteria growth
J Dairy Sci 1999 Nov;82(11):2308-14 Increase of intestinal Bifidobacterium and suppression of coliform bacteria with short-term yogurt ingestion. Chen RM, Wu JJ, Lee SC, Huang AH, Wu HM. Department of Pathology, National Cheng Kung University Medical College, Tainan, Taiwan, Republic of China.PMID: 10575598

Klin Padiatr 1976 Jul;188(4):297-310 [The protective effect of human milk against infections and its potential causes Braun OH. PMID: 824495

Reduces damaging effects of pathogenic bacteria
J Appl Microbiol 1999 Feb;86(2):331-6 Protective effect of bifidus milk on the experimental infection with Salmonella enteritidis subsp. typhimurium in conventional and gnotobiotic mice. Silva AM, Bambirra EA, Oliveira AL, Souza PP, Gomes DA, Vieira EC, Nicoli JR. Departamento de Microbiologia, Faculdade de Medicina, Universidade Federal de Minas Gerais, Belo Horizonte, Brazil. PMID: 10063632

Dig Dis Sci 1997 Nov;42(11):2370-7 Modification of colonic fermentation by bifidobacteria and pH in vitro. Impact on lactose metabolism, short-chain fatty acid, and lactate production. Jiang T, Savaiano DA. Department of Pediatrics, University of Iowa Hospitals and Clinics, Iowa City 52242, USA. PMID: 9398819

Reduces LDL cholesterol
J Dairy Res 1997 Aug;64(3):453-7 Effect of yogurt and bifidus yogurt fortified with skim milk powder, condensed whey and lactose-hydrolysed condensed whey on serum cholesterol and triacylglycerol levels in rats. Beena A, Prasad V. Department of Dairy Science, Veterinary College, Kerala, India. PMID: 9275259

LACTOBACILLUS RHAMNOSUS

Improves bowel movement regularity
Eur J Gastroenterol Hepatol 2001 Apr;13(4):391-6 Results of a double-blind, randomized study to evaluate the efficacy and safety of Antibiophilus in patients with radiation-induced diarrhea. Urbancsek H, Kazar T, Mezes I, Neumann K. Department of Radio-Oncology, Debrecen University Hospital, Nagyerdei krt. 98, H-4032 Debrecen, Hungary. PMID: 11338068

Removes common food carcinogen Aflatoxin B1
J Dairy Sci 2001 Oct;84(10):2152-6 Aflatoxin B1 binding by dairy strains of lactic acid bacteria and bifidobacteria. Peltonen K, el-Nezami H, Haskard C, Ahokas J, Salminen S. Key Centre for Applied and Nutritional Toxicology, School of Medical Sciences, RMIT-University, Buundoora, Victoria 3083, Australia. karita.peltonen@helsinki.fi PMID: 11699445

Appl Environ Microbiol 2001 Jul;67(7):3086-91 Surface binding of aflatoxin B(1) by lactic acid bacteria. Haskard CA, El-Nezami HS, Kankaanpaa PE, Salminen S, Ahokas JT. Key Centre for Applied and Nutritional Toxicology, School of Medical Sciences, RMIT-University, Bundoora, Victoria 3083, Australia. carolyn.haskard@sawater.sa.gov.au PMID: 11425726

Stimulates protective nitrous oxide in immune system and treats viral and antibiotic related diarrhea

Inflammation 2001 Aug;25(4):223-32 Induction of nitric oxide synthesis by probiotic Lactobacillus rhamnosus GG in J774 macrophages and human T84 intestinal epithelial cells. Korhonen R, Korpela R, Saxelin M, Maki M, Kankaanranta H, Moilanen E. The Immunopharmacological Research Group, Medical School, University of Tampere, Finland. PMID: 11580098

Reduces invasiveness of and inhibits toxic E. coli

Int J Food Microbiol 2001 Aug 5;67(3):207-16 In vitro adherence properties of Lactobacillus rhamnosus DR20 and Bifidobacterium lactis DR10 strains and their antagonistic activity against an enterotoxigenic Escherichia coli. Gopal PK, Prasad J, Smart J, Gill HS. New Zealand Dairy Research Institute, Palmerston North. pramod.gopal@nzdri.org.nz PMID: 11518430

Prevents growth of pathogens in gastrointestinal system

Res Microbiol 2001 Mar;152(2):167-73 Probiotic activities of Lactobacillus casei rhamnosus: in vitro adherence to intestinal cells and antimicrobial properties. Forestier C, De Champs C, Vatoux C, Joly B. Laboratoire de bacteriologie, Universite d'Auvergne-Clermont 1, Facultes de medecine-pharmacie, Clermont-Ferrand, France. Christiane.forestier@u-clermont1.fr PMID: 11316370

Prevents rotavirus diarrhea

Clin Diagn Lab Immunol 2001 Mar;8(2):293-6 Adherence of probiotic bacteria to human intestinal mucus in healthy infants and during rotavirus infection. Juntunen M, Kirjavainen PV, Ouwehand AC, Salminen SJ, Isolauri E. Department of Pediatrics, Satakunta Central Hospital, Pori, FIN-25800 Pori, Finland. marketta.juntunen@satshp.fi PMID: 11238211

Enhances immune functioning, natural killer cell activity, and anti-tumor capability by 101-147%

J Clin Immunol 2001 Jul;21(4):264-71 Dietary probiotic supplementation enhances natural killer cell activity in the elderly: an investigation of age-related immunological changes. Gill HS, Rutherfurd KJ, Cross ML. Milk & Health Research Centre, Institute of Food, Nutrition and Human Health, Massey University, Palmerston North, New Zealand. H.S.Gill@massey.ac.nz PMID: 11506196

J Am Coll Nutr 2001 Apr;20(2 Suppl):149-56 Systemic immunity-enhancing effects in healthy subjects following dietary consumption of the lactic acid bacterium Lactobacillus rhamnosus HN001. Sheih YH, Chiang BL, Wang LH, Liao CK, Gill HS. Taipei Medical College Hospital, College of Medicine, National University of Taiwan.PMID: 11349938

REFERENCES

Introduction

Food and Agriculture Organization of the Untied Nations Rome 1999 Fermented Cereals A Global Perspective. Haard N, Odunfa SA, Lee C, Quintero-Ramirez R, Lorence-Quiñones A, Wacher-Radarte C. ISBN 92-5-104296-9

Annals of Medicine 1990 Feb; 22 (1):37-41. Lactic acid bacteria and human health. Gorbach SL. Department of Community Health, Tufts University School of Medicine, Boston, MA

Chapter One
The Miracle of Life

Reuters 2001 September Study Shows Coffee Is Rich Source of Antioxidants. London

Int J Food Microbiol 2001 Jul 20;67(1-2):115-22 Utilization at high pH of starter cultures of lactobacilli for Spanish-style green olive fermentation. Sanchez AH, Rejano L, Montano A, de Castro A. Instituto de la Grasa (CSIC), Padre Garcia Tejero 4, Seville, Spain. PMID: 11482559

J Agric Food Chem 2000 Dec;48(12):5975-80 Comparative study on chemical changes in olive juice and brine during green olive fermentation. Sanchez AH, de Castro A, Rejano L, Montano A. Instituto de la Grasa (CSIC), Apartado 1078, 41012 Seville, Spain. PMID: 11141267

J Food Prot 2000 Jan;63(1):111-6 Content of bigenic amines in table olives. Garcia-Garci P, Brenes-Balbuena M, Hornero-Mendez D, Garcia-Borrego A, Garrido-Fernandez A. Food Biotechnology Department, Instituto de la Grasa (CSIC), Seville, Spain. PMID:10643779

Int J Food Microbiol 1999 Oct 15;51(2-3):133-43 Establishment of conditions for green table olive fermentation at low temperature. Duran Quintana MC, Garcia Garcia P, Garrido Fernandez A. Departamento de Biotecnologia de Alimentos Instituto de la Grasa (CSIC), Seville, Spain. PMID: 10574089

FEBS Lett 1999 June; 452 (1-2):57-60. Mitochondrial assembly in yeast. Grivell LA, Artal-Sanz M, Hakkaart G, de Jong L, Nijtmans LG, van Oosterum K, Siep M, van der Spek H. Section for Molecular Biology, Institute of Molecular Cell Biology, Uni-versity of Amsterdam, The Netherlands. PMID: 10376678

Nutr Rev. 1999 Apr; 57 (4): 114-23. Iron transport across biologic membranes. Andrews NC, Fleming MD, Gunshin H. Howard Hughes Medical Institute, Children's Hospital, Boston, MA. PMID: 10228348

Appl Microbiol Biotechnol 1999 Feb;51(2):249-54 Influence of environmental factors on lipase production by Lactobacillus plantarum. Lopes MD, Cunha AE, Clemente JJ, Carrondo MJ, Crespo MT. Instituto de Biologia Experimental e Tecnologica (IBET)/ Instituto de Tecnologia Quimica e Bilogica (ITQB), Oeiras, Portugal. PMID: 10091332

Int J Food Microbiol 1998 Aug 18;43(1-2):129-34 Bacteriocin production and competitiveness of Lactobacillus plantarum :PCO10 in olive juice broth, a culture medium obtained from olives. Leal MV, Baras M, Ruiz-Barba JL, Floriano B, Jimenez-Diaz R. Departamento de Biotecnologia de Alimentos, Instituto de la Grasa (CSIC), Seville, Spain. PMID: 9761347

J Appl Bacteriol 1994 Apr;76(4):350-5 Vitamin and amino acid requirements of Lacto-bacillus plantarum strains isolated from green olive fermentations. Ruiz-Barba JL, Jimenez-Diaz R. Instituto de la Grasa y sus Derivados (CSIC), Unidad Estructural de Investigacion de Biotecnologia de Alimentos, Seville, Spain. PMID: 8200862

Nahrung 1993;37(3):226-33 Apparent digestibility of dietary fibre and other compo-nents in table olives. Heredia A, Ruiz-Gutierrez V, Felizon B, Guillen R, Jimenez A, Fernandez-Bolanos J. Instituto de la Grasa y sus Derivados (CSIC), Sevilla, Spain. PMID: 8395658

Nahrung 1993;37(6):583-91 Biochemical changes during the preservation stage of ripe olive processing. Garrido A, Garcia P, Montano A, Brenes M, Duran MC. Unidad Estructural de Biotechnologia de Alimentos, Instituto de la Grasa y sus Derivados, (CSIC), Sevilla, Spain. PMID: 8121471

J Appl Bacteriol 1991Nov;71(5):417-21 Plasmid profiles and curing of plasmids in Lactobacillus plantarum strains isolated from green olive fermentations. Ruiz-Barba JL, Piard JC, Jimenez-Diaz R. Instituto de la Grasa y sus Derivados (CSIC), UEI de Biotecnologia de Alimentos, Sevilla, Spain. PMID: 1761434

Can J Microbiol 1978 Jun;24(6):680-4 Utilization of oleuropein by microorganism as-sociated with olive fermentations. Garrido-Fernandez A, Vaughn RH. PMID: 667735

Chapter Two
World Cultures

Curr Microbiol 2002 Jan;44(1):10-7 Characterization of Anti-Listerie monocytogenes Bacteriocins from Enterococcus faecalis, Enterococcus faecium, and Lactococcus lactis Strains Isolated from Raib, a Moroccan Traditional Fermented Milk. Elotmani F, Revol-Junelles AM, Assobhei O, Milliere JB. Laboratoire de Microbiologie Appliquee et Biotechnologie, Faculte des Sciences, Universite Chouaib Doukkali, B.P. 20, 24000 El Jadida, Maroc. PMID: 11727035

Int J Food Microbiol 2001 Feb 28;64(1-2): 193-8 Detection and preliminary character-ization of a bacteriocins (plantaricin 35d) produce by a Lactobacillus plantarum strain. Messi P, Bondi M, Sabia C, Battini R, Manicardi G. Department of Biomedical Sci-ences, University of Medena and Reggio E., Italy. messi.patrizia@unimo.it PMID: 11252503

Mol Microbiol 2000 Aug;37(3):619-28 Functional analysis of promoters involved in quorum sensing-based regulation of bacteriocin production in Lactobacillus. Risoen PA, Brurberg MB, Eijsink VG, Nes IF. Department of Chemistry and Biotechnology, Agricultural University of Norway, N-1432 As, Norway. PMID:10931355

World Health Organization 2000 June 4; WHO Issues New Healthy Life Expectancy Rankings. Press Release, Washington, D.C. and Geneva, Switzerland.

J Appl Microbiol 2000 Jan;88(1):44-51 Bacteriocin production by lactic acid bacteria isolated from Rioja red wines. Navarro L, Zarazaga M, Saenz J, Ruiz-Larrea F, Torres C. Departmento de Agricultura y Alimentacion, Universidad de la Rioja, Logrono, Spain. PMID: 10735242

Food and Agriculture Organization of the Untied Nations Rome 1999 Fermented Cere-als A Global Perspective. Haard N, Odunfa SA, Lee C, Quintero-Ramirez R, Lorence-Quiñones A, Wacher-Radarte C. ISBN 92-5-104296-9

Int J Food Microbiol 1998 Aug 18;43(1-2):129-34 Bacteriocin production and competitiveness of Lactobacillus plantarum LPCO10 in olive juice broth, a culture medium obtained from olives. Leal MV, Baras M, Ruiz-Barba JL, Floriano B, Jimenez-Diaz R. Departamento de Biotecnologia de Alimentos, Instituto de la Grasa (CSIC), Sevilla, Spain. PMID: 9761347

Appl Environ Microbiol 1998 Jun;64(6):2269-72 Antagonistic activity of Lactobacillus plantarum C11: two new two-peptide bacteriocins, plantaricins EF and JK, and the induction factor plantaricin A. Anerssen EL, Diep DB, Nes IF, Eijsink VG, Nissen-Meyer J. Department of Biochemistry, University of Oslo, Oslo, Norway. PMID: 9603847

Int J Food Microbiol 1998 March 3;40(1-2):17-25 Plantaricin LP84, a broad spectrum heat-stable bacteriocins of lactobacillus plantarum NCIM 2084 produced in a simple glucose broth medium. Suma K, Misra MC, Varadaraj MC.Fermentation Technology, Central Food Technological Research Institute, Mysore, India. PMID: 9600606

Antonie Van Leeuwenhoek 1996 Oct;70(2-4):113-28 Biosynthesis of bacteriocins in lactic acid bacteria. New IF, Diep DB, Havarstein LS, Brurberg MB, Eijsinnk V, Holo H. Department of Biotechnological Sciences, Agricultural University of Norway, as, Norway. PMID: 8879403

Biosci Biotechnol Biochem 1994 Nov;58(11):2084-6 Plasmid-associated bacteriocins production by a Lactobacillus plantarum strain. Kanatani K, Oshimura M. Research Laboratory, Tamon Sake Brewing Co., Ltd., Hyogo, Japan. PMID: 7765600

Folia Microbiol (Praha)1994;39(3):181-6 Plasmid profiles of bacteriocins-producing Lactobacillus isolates from African fermented foods. Olasupo NA, Olukoya DK, Odunfa SA. Department of Botany and Microbiology, Faculty of Science, Lagos State University, Ojo, Nigeria. PMID: 7995600

Gut 1997 Jan;40(1):49-56 Alcoholic beverages produced by alcoholic fermentation but not by distillation are powerful stimulants of gastric acid secretion in humans. Teyssen S, Lenzing T, Gonzalez-Calero G, Korn A, Riepl RL, Singer MV. Department of Medicine IV (Gastroenterology), University Hospital of Heidelberg at Mannheim, Germany, <Gut.bmjjournals.com>.

Chapter Three
The Medical Benefits of Culturing
CULTURING

J Pediatr Gastroenterol Nutr 2001 Sep;33(3):307-13 Effect of feeding yogurt versus milk in children with acute diarrhea and carbohydrate malabsorption. Boudraa G, Benbouabdella M, Hachelaf W, Boisset M, Desjeux JF, Touhami M. Service de Pediatrie "c", Amilcar Cabral Clinic, Oran, Algerie; Conservatoire National des Arts et Metiers, Chaire de Biologie, Paris, France. PMID: 11593127

Wire 2001 September 28: Yogurt, Fermented Drinks Good for Bowel Disease. Bitomsky M.

Biosci Biotechnol Biochem 2001 Aug;56(8):1864-8 Prevention by lactic acid bacteria of the oxidation of human LDL.Terahara M Kurama S, Takemoto N. Food Functionality Research Institute, Meiji Milk Products Co., Ltd., Higashimurayama, Toyoko, Japan. PMID: 11577730

Microbial Ecology in Health and Disease 2001 13.(4) 217-222 A fermented milk with a bifidobacterium probiotic strain DN-173 010 Shortened orofecal gut transit time in elderly. Meance S; Gayuela C; Turchet P; Raimondi A; Lucas C; Antoine J (Taylor and Francis Ltd)

J Nutr Sci Vitaminol (Tokyo) 2001 Jun;47(3):253-7 Effect of dietary cabbage fermentation extract and young barley leaf powder on immune function of Sprague-Dawley rats. Mizazaki Y, Tokunaga Y, Takagaki K, Tsusaki S, Tachibana H, Yamada K. Department of Bioscience and Biotechnology, Faculty of Agriculture, Kyushu University, Fukuoka, Japan.PMID: 11575582

J Ind Microbiol Biotehnol 2001 Jun;26(6):327-32 beta-Carotene production in sugarcane molasses by a Rhodotorula glutinis mutant. Bhosale P, Gadre RV. Chemical Engineering division, National Chemical Laboratory, Pune 411 008, India. PMID: 11571614

Int Immunopharmacol 2001 May; 1 (5):891-901 Anti-allergy properties of fermented foods: an important immunoregulatory mechanism of lactic acid bacteria? Cross ML, Stevenson LM, Gill HS. Milk and Health Research Centre, Institute of Food, Nutrition and Human Health, Massey University, Palmerston North, New Zealand. PMID: 11379044

J Altern Complement Med 2001 Apr;7(2):133-9 An analysis of nine proprietary Chinese red yeast rice dietary supplements: implications of variability in chemical profile and contents. Heber D, Lembertas A, Lu QY, Bowerman S, Go VL. UCLA Center for Human Nutrition, UCLA School of Medicine, Los Angeles, California 90095-1742, USA. dheber@mednet.ucla.edu PMID: 11327519

Am J Clin Nutr 2001 Feb; 73 (2 Suppl):451S-455S Protective role of probiotics and prebiotics in colon cancer. Wollowski I, Rechkemmer G, Pool-Zobel BL. Institute for Nutritional Physiology, Federal Research Centre for Nutrition, Karlsruhe, Germany. PMID: 11157356

J Nutr 2001 Jan;131(1):111-7 Food supplementation with milk fermented by Lactobacillus casei DN-114 001 protects suckling rats from rotavirus-associated diarrhea. Guerin-Dana C, Meslin JC, Chambard A, Charpilienne A, Relano P, Bouley C, Cohen J, Andrieux C. INRA, UEPSD, MBS, 78352 Jouy en Josas cedex, France PMID: 11208946

Biosci Biotechnol Biochem 2000 Dec; 64 (12):2706-8 Effects of a fermented milk drink containing Lactobacillus casei strain Shirota on the immune system in healthy human subjects. Nagao F, Nakayama M, Muto T, Okumura K. PMID: 11210142

Int J food Microbiol 2000 Sep 25;60(2-3):163-9 In vitro digestibility of bacillus fermented soya bean. Kiers JL, Van Laeken AE, Rombouts FM, Nout MJ. Wageningen University, Agrotechnology and Food Sciences, Laboratory of Food Microbiology, The Netherlands. jcrocn.kicrs@micro.fdsci.wag-ur.nl PMID: 11016606

Biosci Biotechnol Biochem 2000 May;64(5):1038-40 1, 1-Diphenyl-2-picrylhydrazyl radical-scavenging compounds from soybean miso and antiproliferative activity of isoflavones from soybean miso toward the cancer cell lines. Hirota A, Taki S, Kawaii S, Yano M, Abe N. Laboratory of Applied Microbiology, School of Food and Nutritional Sciences, University of Shizuoka, Japan. hirotaa@u-shizuoka-ken.ac.jp PMID: 10879475

Carcinogenesis 2000 May;21(5):937-41 Inhibitory effects of Bifidobacterium-fermented soy milk on 2-amino-1-methyl-6-phenylimidazo[4,5-b]pyridine-induced rat mammary carcinogenesis, with a partial contribution of its component isoflavones. Ohta T, Nakatsugi S, Watanabe K, Kawamori T, Ishikawa F, Morotomi M, Sugie S, Toda T, Sugimura T, Wakabayashi K. Cancer Prevention Division, National Cancer Center Research Institute, 1-1 Tsukiji 5-chome, Chuo-ku, Tokyo, Japan. PMID:10783315

Nahrung 2000 Apr;44(2):85-8 Tarhana as a traditional Turkish fermented cereal food. Its recipe, production and composition. Daglioglu O. Department of Food Engineering, Trakya University, Agriculture Faculty of Tekirdag, Turkey. PMID: 10795573

J Agric Fod Chem 2000 Apr;48(4):1367-72 Soybean meal fermented by Aspergillus awamori increases the cytochrome P-450 content of the liver microsomes of mice. Kishida T, Ataki H, Takebe N, Ebihara K. Department of Biological Resources, Faculty of Agriculture, Ehime University, 3-5-7 Tarumi, Matsuyama 790-8566, Japan. PMID: 10775399

Am J Gastroenterol 2000 Apr;95(4):1017-20 Fermentation of dietary starch in humans. Ahmed R, Segal I, Hassan H. Gastroenterology Division, Chris Hani Baragwanath Hospital, Soweto, South Africa. PMID: 10763953

Biosci Biotechnol Biochem 2000 Mar;64(3):617-9 Changes in gamma-aminobutyric acid content during beni-koji making. Kono I, Himeno K. Industrial Technology Center of Okayama Prefecture, Okayama-shi, Japan. PMID: 10803966

Free Radic Biol Med 2000 Mar 15;28(6):999-1004 Dimerumic acid as an antioxidant of the mold, Monascus anka. Aniya Y, Ohtani II, Higa T, Miyagi C, Gibo H, Shimabukuro M, Nakanishi H, Taira J. Laboratory of Physiology and Pharmacology, School of Health Sciences, Faculty of Medicine, University of the Ryukyus, Okinawa, Japan. Yaniya@med.u-ryukyu.ac.jp PMID: 10802232

J Food Prot 2000 Mar;63(3):364-9 Inhibitory power of kefir: the role of organic acids. Garrote GL, Abraham AG, De Antoni GL. Centro de Investigacion y Desarrollo en Criotecnologia de Alimentos, La Plata, Argentina. PMID: 10716566

Am J Clin Nutr 2000 Mar;7193):674-81 Consumption of fermented and nonfermented dairy products: effects on cholesterol concentrations and metabolism St- Onge MP, Farnworth ER, Jones PJ. School of Dietetics and Human Nutrition, McGill University, Ste-Anne-de-Bellevue, Canada. PMID: 10702159

Biosci Biotechnol Biochem 2000 Feb;64(2):414-6 Antimutagenicity of the purple pigment, hordeumin, from uncooked barley bran-fermented broth. Deguchi T, Yoshimoto M, Ohba R, Ueda S, Department of Applied Microbial Technology, Faculty of Engineering, Kumamoto Institute of Technology, Japan. PMID: 10737202

J Bone Miner Metab 2000;18(2):71-6 Prolonged intake of fermented soybean (natto) diets containing vitamin K2 (menaquinone-7) prevents bone loss in ovariectomized rats. Yamaguchi M, Kakuda H, Gao YH, Tsukamoto Y. Laboratory of Endocrinology and Molecular Metabolism, Graduate School of Nutritional Sciences, University of Shizuoka, Japan. PMID: 10701161

Crit Rev Biotechnol 2000;20(4):265-91 Control of foodborne pathogens during sufu fermentation and aging. Shi Xj, Fung Dy. Department of Animal Sciences and Industry, Kansas State University, Manhattan, KS 66506-1600, USA. PMID: 11192025

J Bone Miner Metab 2000;18(4):216-22 Intake of fermented soybean (natto) increases circulating vitamin K2 (menaquinone-7) and gamma-carboxylated osteocalcin concentration in normal individuals. Tsukamoto Y, Ichise H, Kakuda H, Yamaguchi M. Central Research Institute, Mitsukan group Co., Ltd., Aichi, Japan. PMID: 10874601

Appl Environ Microbiol 1999 Nov;65(11):4725-8 Antiproliferative effects of homogenates derived from five strains of candidate probiotic bacteria.Pessi T, Sutas Y, Saxelin M, Kallioinen H, Isolauri E. Department of Pediatrics, University of Turku, Turku, Finland. tanja.pessi@valio.fi PMID: 10543777

138

Int J food Sci Nutr 1999 Nov;50(6):451-5 Survival of some species of Salmonella and Shigella in mukumbi, a traditional Zimbabwean wine. Mugochi T, Parawira W, Mpofu A, Simango C, Zvauya R. Department of Biochemistry, University of Zimbabwe, Harare. PMID: 10719586

Biosci Biotechnol Biochem 1999 Sep;63(9):1637-9 New potent antioxidative o-dihydroxyisoflavones in fermented Japanese soybean products. Esaki H, Kawakishi S, Morimitsu Y, Osawa T, Department of Food and Nutrition, Sugiyama Jogakuen Univerisity, Nagoya, Japan. PMID: 10540753

Plant Foods Hum Nutr 1999;53(2):103-11 Reduction of some toxicants in Icacina mannii by fermentation with Saccharomyces cerevisiae. Antai SP, Nkwelang G. Department of Biological Sciences, University of Calabar, Nigeria PMID: 10472787

J Ethnopharmacol 1999 Jul; 66 (1):11-7. Antioxidant and eicosanoid enzyme inhibition properties of pomegranate seed oil and fermented juice flavonoids. Schubert SY, Lansky EP, Neeman I. Laboratories of Food Engineering and Biotechnology, Technion-Israel Institute of Technology, Haifa. PMID: 10432202

Int J Clin Pract 1999 Apr-May;53(3):179-84 The effect of supplementation with milk fermented by Lactobacillus casei (strain DN-114 001) on acute diarrhea in children attending day care centres. Pedone CA, Bernabeu AO, Postaire ER, Bouley CF, Reinert P. CIRDC (Centre International de Recherche Daniel Carasso), groupe Santé-Nutrition, Le Plessis Robinson, France. PMID: 10665128

J Am Coll Nutr 1999 Feb; 18 (1):43-50. Effect of fermented milk (yogurt) containing Lactobacillus acidophilus L1 on serum cholesterol in hypercholesterolemic humans. Anderson JW, Gilliland SE. Metabolic Research Group, VA Medical Center, University of Kentucky, Lexington. PMID: 10067658

J Agric Food Chem 1999 Feb;47(2):363-71 Characteristics and use of okara, the soybean residue from soy milk production –a review. O'Toole DK. Bioactive Products Research Group, Department of Biology and Chemistry, City University of Hong Kong, Kowloon, China. bhsnuff@cityu.edu.hk PMID: 10563901

Nutrition 1998 Oct; 14 (10):763-766. Complimentary feeding: a global perspective. Michaelsen KF, Friis H. Research Department of Human Nutrition, Royal Veterinary and Agricultural University, Frederiksberg, Denmark. kfm@kvl.dk PMID: 9785357

Int J Food Microbiol 1998 Jun; 42 (1-2):29-38. Survival of Lactobacillus plantarum DSM 9843 (299v), and effect on the short-chain fatty acid content of faeces after ingestion of a rose-hip drink with fermented oats. Johansson ML, Noback S, Berggren A, Nyman M, Bjorck I, Ahrne S, Jeppsson B, Molin G. Probi AB, Ideon Gamma 1, Lund, Sweden. marie.louise@probi.ideon.se. PMID: 9706795

Biochem Mol Biol Int 1998 Jun; 45 (1):11-23. Free radical scavenging activity of fermented papaya preparation and its effect on lipid peroxide level and superoxide dismutase activity in iron-induced epileptic foci of rats. Imao K, Wang H, Komatsu M, Hiramatsu M. SAIDO Co., Fukuoka, Japan. PMID: 9635126

Jpn J Cancer Res 1998 May; 89 (5):487-95. Chemoprevention of N-nitroso-N-methylurea-induced rat mammary cancer by miso and tamoxifen, alone and in combination. Gotoh T, Yamada K, Ito A, Yin H, Kataoka T, Dohi K. Department of Cancer Research, Hiroshima University. PMID: 9685851

J Dairy Sci 1998 May; 81 (5):1229-35. Cell-free whey from milk fermented with Bifidobacterium breve C50 used to modify the colonic microflora of healthy subjects. Romond MB, Ais A, Guillemot F, Bounouader R, Cortot A, Romond C. Laboratoire de Bacteriologie, Faculté des Sciences Pharmaceutiques et Biologiques, Lille, France. PMID: 9621224

Nutr Cancer 1998; 32 (1):25-8. Effects of miso and NaCl on the development of colonic aberrant crypt foci induced by azoxymethane in F344 rats. Masaoka Y, Watanabe H, Katoh O, Ito A, Dohi K. Department of Environment and Mutation, Hiroshima University, Japan. PMID: 9824853

Dairy Res 1998 Feb; 65 (1);129-38. Antitumour activity of yogurt: study of possible immune mechanisms. Perdigon G, Valdez JC, Rachid M. Instituto de Microbiologia, Facultad de Bioquimica, Quimica y Farmacia, Universidad Nacional de Tucuman, Argentina. PMID: 9513059

Am J Cardiol 1997 Dec; 80 (12):1627-31. Inhibition of human low-density lipopro-tein oxidation by flavonoids in red wine and grape juice. Miyagi Y, Miwa K, Inoue H. The Department of Cardiology, Rakuwakai Otowa Hospital, Kyoto, Japan. PMID: 9416955

Coron Artery Dis 1997 Oct; 8 (10):645-9. Alcohol, ischemic heart desease, and the French paradox. Constant J. State University of New York at Buffalo. PMID: 9457446

Cell Growth Differ 1997 May; 8 (5):523-32. Short-chain fatty acid-initiated cell cycle arrest and apoptosis of colonic epithelial cells is linked to mitochondrial function. Heerdt BG, Houston MA, Augenlicht LH. Albert Einstein Cancer Center, Bronx, New York 10467, USA. PMID: 9149903

J Nutr Sci Vitaminol 1997 Apr; 42 (2):249-59. Antioxidative mechanism and apoptosis induction by 3-hydroxyanthranilic acid, an antioxidant in Indonesian food Tempeh, in the human hepatoma-derived cell line, HuH-7. Matsuo M, Nakamura N, Shidoji Y, Muto Y, Esaki H, Osawa T. Gifu Women's University, Japan. PMID: 9219098

Nutr Cancer 1997; 28 (1):93-97. Antiproliferative effect of fermented milk on the growth of a human breast cancer cell line. Biffi A, Coradini D, Larsen R, Riva L, Di Fronzo G. Istituto Nazionale per lo Studio e la Cura dei Tumori, Milan, Italy. PMID: 9200156

Nutr Cancer 1997; 29 (3):228-33. Decreased serum estradiol concentration associ-ated with high dietary intake of soy products in premenopausal Japanese women. Nagata C, Kabuto M, Kurisu Y, Shimizu H. Department of Public Health, Gifu Uni-versity School of Medicine, Japan. chisato@cc.gifu-u.ac.jp. PMID: 9457744

Biofactors 1997; 6 (4):403-10. Polyphenols produced during red wine ageing. Brouillard R, George F, Fougerousse A. Laboratoire de Chimie des Polyphenols, Université Louis Pasteur, Faculté de Chimie, Strasbourg, France. PMID: 9388306

J Nutr 1996 Dec; 126 (12):3063-8. Antihypertensive peptides are present in aorta after oral administration of sour milk containing these peptides to spontaneously hy-pertensive rats. Masuda O, Nakamura Y, Takano T. R&D Center, The Calpis Food Industry Co., Ltd., Fuchinobe, Sagamirara, Japan. PMID: 9001375

Am J Clin Nutr 1996 Nov; 64 (5):767-71. A placebo-controlled study of the effect of sour milk on blood pressure in hypertensive subjects. Hata Y, Yamamoto M, Ohni M, Nakajima K, Nakamura Y, Takano T. Department of Medicine and Gerontology, Kyorin University School of Medicine, Tokyo, Japan. PMID: 8901799

J Dairy Sci 1996 May; 79 (5):745-9. Effect of administration of milk fermented with Lactobacillus acidophilus LA-2 on fecal mutagenicity and microflora in the human intestine. Hosoda M, Hashimoto H, He F, Morita H, Hosono A. Technical Research Laboratory, Takanashi Milk Products Co., LTD, Yokohama, Japan. PMID: 8792276

Food Chem Toxicol 1996 May; 34 (5):457-61. Quantification of genistein and genistin in soybeans and soybean products. Fukutake M, Takahashi M, Ishida K, Kawamura H, Sugimura T, Wakabayashi K. Biochemistry Division, National Cancer Center Research Institute, Tokyo, Japan. PMID: 8655094

Alt Med Rev 1996;194):258-274 Phosphatidylcholine: A Superior Protectant Against Liver Damage Parris M. Kidd, Ph.D.

Mutat Res 1996 Feb; 350 (1):199-200. Antimutagenicity of yogurt. Bakalinsky AT, Nadathur SR, Carney JR, Gould SJ. Department of Food Science and Technology, Oregon State University, Corvallis. PMID: 8657181

J Basic Microbiol 1995;35(5):319-24 Studies on bacteriocinogenic Lactobacillus isolates from selected Nigerian fermented foods. Olasupo NA, Olukoya DK, Odunfa SA. Department of Botany and Microbiology, Faculty of Science, Lagos State University, Ojo, Nigeria. PMID: 8568643

J Dairy Sci 1995 Jul; 78 (7):1597-606. Immune system stimulation by probiotics. Perdigon G, Alvarez S, Rachid M, Aguero G, Gobbato N. Centro de Referencias para Lactobacilos (CERELA), Tucuman, Argentina. PMID: 7593855

J of the American Diet Assoc 1995 May; 95 (5):545-51. Urinary isoflavonoid phytoestrogen and lignan excretion after consumption of fermented and unfermented soy products. Hutchins AM, Slavin JL, Lampe JW. Department of Food Science and Nutrition, University of Minnesota, St. Paul. PMID: 7722188

Mutat Res 1995 Apr; 334 (2):213-24. Antimutagenicity of an acetone extract of yogurt. Nadathur SR, Gould SJ, Bakalinsky AT. Department of Food Science and Technology, Oregon State University, Corvallis. PMID: 7885375

Carcinogenesis 1995 Mar; 13 (3):471-6. Possible anti-tumour-promoting activity of components in Japanese soybean fermented food, Natto: effect of gap junctional intercellular communication. Takahashi C, Kikuchi N, Katou N, Miki T, Yanagida F, Umeda M. Department of Brewing and Fermentation, Faculty of Agriculture, Tokyo University of Agriculture, Japan. PMID: 7697800

J Pediatr Gastroenterol Nutr 1995 Feb; 20 (2):189-95. Prospective study of lactose absorption during cancer chemotherapy: feasibility of a yogurt-supplemented diet in lactose malabsorbers. Pettoello-Mantovani M, Guandalini S, diMartino L, Corvino C, Indolfi P, Casale F, Giuliano M, Dubrovsky L, Di Tullio MT. Department of Pediatrics, University of Naples, Italy. PMID: 95230453

Plant Foods for Human Nut 1995 Jan; 47 (1):39-47. Anti-hypertensive substances in fermented soybean, natto. Okamoto A, Hanagata H, Kawamura Y, Yanagida F. Department of Brewing and Fermentation, Tokyo University of Agriculture, Japan. PMID: 7784396

J Nutr Sci Vitaminol 1994 Dec; 40 (6):613-6. Effect of Lactobacillus acidophilus on iron bioavailability in rats. Oda T, Kado-Oka Y, Hashiba H. Technical Research Institute, Snow Brand Milk Products Co. Ltd., Kawagoe, Japan. PMID: 7751979

141

J Nutr Sci Vitaminol 1994 Oct; 40 (5):467-77. Antioxidative effects of a processed grain food. Minamiyama Y, Yoshikawa T, Tanigawa T, Takahashi S, Naito Y, Ichikawa H, Kondo M. First Department of Internal Medicine, Kyoto Prefectural University of Medicine, Japan. PMID: 7891207

Zeitschrift Für Lebensmittel-Untersuchung Und-Forschung 1994 Mar; 198 (3):193-201. The potential of lactic acid bacteria for the production of safe and wholesome food. Hammes WP, Tichaczek PS. Institut für Lebensmitteltechnologie, Universität Hohenheim, Stuttgart, Germany. PMID: 8178575

Mutat Res 1993 Aug; 300 (3-4):201-6. Anticlastogenic and bio-antimutagenic activ-ity of cultured broth of Saccharomyces cerevisiae 28 on mutagens. Zhang XB, Ohta Y. Labora-tory for Microbial Biochemistry, Faculty of Applied Biological Science, Hiroshima Uni-versity, Higashi, Japan. PMID: 7687019

J Nutr Sci Vitaminol 1992 Jun; 38 (3):297-304. Japanese soybean paste miso scavenges free radicals and inhibits lipid peroxidation. Santiago LA, Hiramatsu M, Mori, A. Depart-ment of Neurochemistry, Okayama University Medical School, Japan. PMID: 1333523

Rocz Panstw Zakl Hig 1992; 43 (3-4):253-8. Effect of the fermentation process on levels of nitrates and nitrites in selected vegetables. Herod-Leszczynska T, Miedzobrodzka A. Zywienia Czlowieka Akademii Rolniczej, Krakowie, Poland. PMID: 1308742

J Dairy Sci 1991 Mar; 74 (3):758-63. Antimicrobial activity of Microgard against food spoilage and pathogenic microorganisms. al-Zoreky N, Ayres JW, Sandine WE. Depart-ment of Food Science and Technology, Oregon State University, Corvallis. PMID: 1906486

J Dairy Sci 1990 Dec; 73 (12):3379-84. Antimutagenic activity of milk fermented by Streptococcus thermophilus and Lactobacillus bulgaricus. Bodana AR, Rao DR. Ala-bama A&M University, Normal 35762. PMID: 2099363

J Pediatr Gastroenterol Nutr 1990 Nov; 11 (4):509-12. Effect of feeding yogurt ver-sus milk in children with persistent diarrhea. Boudraa G, Touhami M, Pochart P, Soltana R, Mary JY, Desjeux JF. Dervice de Pediatrie, C. Oran, Algerie. PMID: 2262840

Dig Dis Sci 1990 May; 35 (5):630-7. In vitro antibacterial effect of yogurt on Es-cherichia coli. Kotz CM, Peterson LR, Moody JA, Savaiano DA, Levitt MD. Re-search Service, Veterans Affairs Medical Center, Minneapolis, MN. PMID: 2185003

Nutr Cancer 1990; 14 (2):103-9. Effect of miso (Japanese soybean paste) and NaCl on DMBA-induced rat mammary tumors. Baggott JE, Ha T Vaughn WH, Juliana MM, Hardin JM, Grubbs CJ. Department of Nutrition Sciences, University of Alabama, Birmingham. PMID:2120681

Chinese J of Prev 1989 Nov; 23 (6):352-4. A study on the effect of fermented soybean in preventing iron deficiency anemia in children. Qin HS. PMID: 2627849

Cancer Res 1989 Jul; 49 (14):4020-3. Consumption of fermented milk products and breast cancer: a case-control study in the Netherlands. Van't Veer P, Dekker JM, Lamers J W, Kok FJ, Schouten EG, Brants HS, Sturmans F, Hermus RJ. Epidemiology Section, TNO_CIVO Toxicology and Nutrition Institute, Zeist, The Netherlands. PMID: 2736542

Indian J Exp Biol 1989 Jan; 24 (1):72-5. Cytotoxic activity of lactobacilli isolated from plant and dairy sources. Manjunath N, Ranganathan B. PMID: 2606525

Clin Radiol 1988 Jul; 39 (4):435-7. Preservation of intestinal integrity during radio-therapy using live Lactobacillus acidophilus cultures. Salminen E, Elomaa I, Minkkinen J, Vapaatalo H, Salminen S. Department of Radiotherapy and Oncology, Helsinki University Hospital, Finland. PMID:3141101

Immunology 1988 Jan; 63 (1):17-23. Systemic augmentation of the immune response in mice by feeding fermented milks with Lactobacillus casei and Lactobacillus acidophilus. Perdigon G, de Macias ME, Alvarez S, Oliver G, de Ruiz Holgado AP. PMID: 3123370

J Dairy Sci 1986 Sep; 69 (9):2237-42. Antimutagenic properties of lactic acid-cultured milk on chemical and fecal mutagens. Hosono A, Kashina T, Kada T, Faculty of Agriculture, Shinshu University, Nagano-Kenya. PMID:3097092

Antonie Van Leeuwenhoek 1983 Sep; 43 (3):337-48. Lactic acid fermentation in the production of foods from vegetables, cereals and legumes. Steinkraus KH. PMID: 6354083

J Dairy Sci 1982 Dec; 65 (12):2388-90. Ion exchange separation of the antitumor component(s) of yogurt dialyzate. Ayebo AD, Shahani KM, Dam R, Friend BA. PMID: 7161436

Nut Biochem & Biotech Improving Nutritional Quality and Hygienic safety in Supplementary Foods for Young Children. Svanberg U. Department of Food Science. Chalmers University of Technology, Gothenburg, Sweden.

Calcif Tissue Int 1992 Mar; 50(3):261-5. Liposome interactions with hydroxyapatite crystals: a possible mechanism in the calcification of atherosclerotic plaques. Hirsch D, Landis WJ Azoury R, Sarig S. Casali Institute of Applied Chemistry, Graduate School of Applied Science and Technology, Hebrew University of Jerusalem, Israel. PMID: 1617501

Nahrung 1987;31 (3):225-32 Proteoulytic activity of crude cell-free extract of Lactobacillus casei and Lactobacillus plantarum. Hegazi FZ, Abo-Elnaga IG. PMID: 3112575

Med Microbiol Immunol (Berl) 1984;173(3):113-25 Comparison of antitumor activity of Lactobacillus casei with other bacterial immunopotentiators. Yasutake N, Ohwaki M, Yokokura T, Mutai M. PMID: 6438456

Biull Eksp Biol Med 1977 Dec;84(12): 709-12 [Antitumor effect of glycopeptides from the cell wall of Lactobacillus bulgaricus.] Bogdanov IG, Velichkov VT, Gurevich AI, Dalev PG, Kolosov MN. PMID:597607

YEAST COFACTORS/PROBIOTIC

Am J Clin Nutr 2001 Feb; 73 (2 Suppl):437S-443S. Probiotic agents to protect the urogenital tract against infection. Reid G. Lawson Research Institute and the Department of Microbiology and Immunology, the University of Western Ontario, Canada. gregor@julian.uwo.com PMID: 11157354

Biosci Biotechnol Biochem 2001 Apr; 65 (4):837-41. Purification of soluble beta-glucan with immune-enhancing activity from the cell wall of yeast. Lee JN, Lee DY, Ji IH, Kim HN, Sohn J, Kim S, Kim CW. Graduate School of Biotechnology, Korea University, Seoul. PMID: 11388461

Eur J Biochem 2001 Apr; 268 (8):2351-61. A subfraction of the yeast endoplasmic reticulum associates with the plasma membrane and has a high capacity to synthesize lipids. Pichler H, Gaigg B, Hrastnik C, Achleitner G, Kohlwein SD, Zellnig G, Perktold A, Daum G. Institut für Biochemie, Technische Universität, and SFB Biomembrane Research Center, Graz, Austria. PMID: 11298754

Enzyme Microb Technol 2000 Jun 1; 26 (9-10):737-742. A short review on the role of glutathione in the response of yeasts to nutritional, environmental, and oxidative stresses. Pennickx M. Laboratoire de Physiologie et Ecologie Microbiennes, Université Libre de Bruxelles c/o IP. 642, Rue Engeland. B-1180 Brussells, Belgium. PMID: 10862879

Mol Microbiol 2000 Feb; 35 (3):477-89. beta-1,6-Glucan synthesis in Saccharomyces cerevisiae. Shahinian S, Bussey H. Department of Biology, McGill University, 1205 Dr Penfield Avenue, Montreal Quebec, Canada. PMID: 10672173

Mikrobiol Z 1999 Nov-Dec; 61 (6):42-50. (Article in Russian) The bacteriocinogenic and lysozyme-synthesizing activity of lactobacilli. Kovalenko NK, Nemirovskaia LN, Kasumova SA. Institute of Microbiology and Virology, National Academy of Sciences of Ulkraine, Kyiv. PMID: 10707532

Crit Rev Food Sci Nutr 1999 Mar; 39 (2):189-202. Effect of beta-glucan from oats and yeast on serum lipids. Bell S, Goldman VM, Bistrian BR, Arnold AH, Ostroff G,Forse RA. Harvard Medical School, Boston, MA. PMID: 10198754

J AM Coll Nutr 1999 Feb; 18 (1):43-50. Effect of fermented milk (yogurt) containing Lactobacillus acidophilus L1 on serum cholesterol in hypercholesterolemic humans. Anderson JW, Gilliland SE. Metabolic Research Group, VA Medical Center, University of Kentucky, Lexington. PMID: 10067658

Int J Food Microbiol 1998 Jun; 42 (1-2):29-38. Survival of Lactobacillus plantarum DSM 9843 (299v), and effect on the short-chain fatty acid content of faeces after ingestion of a rose-hip drink with fermented oats. Johansson ML, Nobaek S, Berggren A, Nyman M, Bjorck I, Ahrne S, Jeppsson B, Molin G, Probi AB, Ideon Gamma L. Lund, Sweden. marie.louise@probi.ideon.se. PMID: 9706795

Jpn J Cancer Res 1998 May; 89 (5):487-95. Chemoprevention of N-nitroso-N-Methylurea- induced rat mammary cancer by miso and tamoxifen, alone and in combination. Gotoh T, Yamada K, Ito A, Yin H, Kataoka T, Dohi K. Department of Cancer Research, Hiroshima University. PMID: 9685851

J Dairy Sci 1998 May; 81 (5):1229-35. Cell-free whey from milk fermented with Bifidobacterium breve C50 used to modify the colonic microflora of heathly subjects. Romond MD, Ais A, Guillemot F, Bounouader R, Cortot A, Romond C. Laboratoire de Bacteriologie, Faculté des Sciences Pharmaceutiques et Biologiques, Lille, France. PMID: 9621224

Int J Food Microbiol 1998 Mar 3; 40 (1-2):17. Plantaricin LP84, a broad spectrum heat-stable bacteriocin of Lactobacillus plantarum NCIM 2084 produced in a simple glucose broth medium. Suma K, Misra MC, Varadaraj MC. Fermentation Technology, Central Food Technological Research Institute, Mysore, India. PMID: 9600606

Dairy Res 1998 Feb; 65 (1):129-38. Antitumour activity of yogurt: study of possible immune mechanisms. Perdigon G, Valdex JC, Rachid M. Intituto de Microbiolagia, Facultad de Bioquimica, Quimica y Farmacia, Universidad Nacional de Tucuman, Argentina. PMID: 9513059

Nutr Cancer 1998; 32 (1):25-8. Effects of miso and NaCl on the development of colonic aberrant crypt foci induced by azoxymethane in F344 rats. Masaoka Y, Watanabe H, Katoh O, Ito A, Dohi K. Department of Environment and Mutation, Hiroshima University, Japan. PMID: 9824853

Am J Cardiol 1997 Dec; 80 (12):1627-31. Inhibition of human low-density lipoprotein oxidation by flavonoids in red wine and grape juice. Miyagi Y, Miwa K, Inoue H. The Department of Cardiology, Rakuwakai Otowa Hospital, Kyoto, Japan. PMID: 9416955

Coron Artery Dis 1997 Oct; 8 (10):645-9. Alcohol, ischemic heart disease, and the French paradox. Constant J. State University of New York at Buffalo. PMID: 9457446

Biosci Biotechnol Biochem 1997 May; 61 (5):884-6. Isolation and partial amino acid sequence of bacteriocins produced by Lactobacillus acidophilus. Tahara T, Kanatani K. Research Laboratory, Tamon Sake Brewing Co., Ltd., Hyogo, Japan. PMID: 9178566

J Nutr Sci Vitaminol 1997 Apr; 43 (2):249-59 Antioxidative mechanism and apoptosis induction by 3-hydroxyanthranilic acid, an antioxidant in Indonesian food Tempeh, in Crit Rev Food Sci Nutr 1999 Mar; 39 (2):189-202. Effect of beta-glucan from oats and yeast on serum lipids. Bell S, Goldman VM, Bistrian BR, Arnold AH, Ostroff G, Forse RA. Harvard Medical School, Boston, MA. PMID: 10198754

J Nutr Sci Vitaminol 1997 Apr; 43 (2):249-59 Antioxidative mechanism and apoptosis induction by 3-hydroxyanthranilic acid, an antioxidant in Indonesian food Tempeh, in the human hepatoma-derived cell line, HuH-7. Matsuo M, Nakamura N, Shidoji Y, Muto Y, Esaki H, Osawa T. Gifu Women's University, Japan. PMID: 9219098

Biofactors 1997; 6 (4):403-10. Polyphenols produced during red wine ageing. Brouillard R, George F, Fougerousse A. Laboratoire de Chimie des Polyphenols, Université Louis Pasteur, Faculté de Chimie, Strasbourg, France. PMID: 9388306

Nutr Cancer 1997; 29 (3):228-33. Decreased serum estradiol concentration associated with high dietary intake of soy products in premenopausal Japanese women. Nagata C, Kabuto M, Kurisu Y, Shimizu H. Department of Public Health, Gifu University School of Medicine, Japan. chisato@cc.gifu-u.ac.jp PMID: 9457744

Nutr Cancer 1997; 28 (1):93-9. Antiproliferative effect of fermented milk on the growth of a human breast cancer cell line. Biffi A, Coradini D, Larsen R, Riva L, Di Fronzo G. Istituto Nazionale per lo Studio e la Cura dei Tumori, Milan, Italy. PMID: 9200156

Am J Clin Nutr 1996 Nov; 64 (5):767-71. A placebo-controlled study of the effect of sour milk on blood pressure in hypertensive subjects. Nakajima K, Nakamura Y, Takano T, Hata Y, Yamamoto M, Ohni M. PMID: 8901799

Food Chem Toxicol 1996 May; 34 (5):457-61. Quantification of genistein and genistin in soybean products. Fukutake M, Takahashi M, Ishida K, Kawamura H, Sugimura T, Wakabayashi K. Biochemistry Division, National Cancer Center Research Institute,Tokyo, Japan. PMID: 8655094

J Dairy Sci 1996 May; 79 (5):745-9. Effect of administration of milk fermented with Lactobacillus acidophilus LA-2 on fecal mutagenicity and microflora in the human intestine. Hosoda M, Hashimoto H, He F, Morita H, Hosono A. Technical Research Laboratory, Takanshi Milk Products Co., Ltd., Yokohama, Japan. PMID: 8792276

FEBS Lett 1995 Jul 10; 368 (1):73-6. Oxidative stress response in yeast: effect of glutathione on adaptation to hydrogen peroxide stress in Saccharomyces cerevisiae. Izawa S, Inoue Y, Kimura A. Research Institute for Food Science, Kyoto University, Japan. PMID: 7615092

J Dairy Sci 1995 Jul; 78 (7):1597-606. Immune system stimulation by probiotics. Perdigon G, Alvarez S, Rachid M, Aguero G, Gobbato N. Centro de Referencias para Lactobacilos (CERELA), Tucuman, Argentina. PMID: 7593855

J of the Amer Diet Assoc 1995 May: 95 (5):545-51. Urinary isoflavonoid phytoestrogen and lignan excretion after consumption of fermented and unfermented soy products. Hutchins AM, Slavin JL, Lampe JW. Department of Food Science and Nutrition, University of Minnesota, St. Paul. PMID: 10744130

Carcinogenesis 1995 Mar; 16 (3):471-6. Possible anti-tumour promoting activity of components in Japanese soybean fermented food, Natto: effect on gap junctional intercellular communication. Takahashi C, Kikuchi N, Katou N, Miki T, Yanagida F, Umeda M. Argentina.

J Pediatr Gastroenterol Nutr 1995 Feb; 20 (2):189-95. Prospective study of lactose absorption during cancer chemotherapy: feasibility of a yogurt-supplemented diet in lactose malabsorbers. Pettoello-Mantovani M, Guandalini S, diMartino L, Corvino C, Indolfi P, Casale F, Giuliano M, Dubrovsky L, Di Tullio MT. Department of Pedi-atrics, University of Naples, Italy. PMID: 7714685

Plant Foods for Human Nutr 1995 Jan; 47 (1):39-47. Anti-hypertensive substances in fermented soybean, natto. Okamoto A, Hanagata H, Kawamura Y, Yanagida F. PMID: 7784396

J Dairy Sci 1993 Aug; 76 (8):2366-79. Antibiosis revisited: bacteriocins produced by dairy starter cultures. Barfoot SF, Nettles CG. Department of Food Science, Clemson University, SC. PMID: 8408870

Mutation Research 1993 Aug; 300 (3-4):201-206. Anticlastongenic and bio-antimu-tagenic activity of cultured broth of Saccharomyces cerevisiae 28 on mutagens. Zhang X, Ohta Y. Laboratory for Microbiol Biochemistry, Faculty of Applied Biological Science, Hiroshima University, Higashi-Hiroshima 724, Japan. PMID: 7687019

J Nutr Sci Vitaminol 1992 Jun; 38 (3)297-304. Japanese soybean paste miso scavenges free radicals and inhibits lipid peroxidation. Santiago LA, Hiramatsu M, Mori A. Department of Neurochemistry, Okayama University Medical School, Japan. PMID:1333523

J Dairy Sci 1990 Dec; 73 (12):3379-84. Antimutagenic activity of milk fermented by Streptococcus thermophilus and Lactobacillus bulgarius. Bodana AR, Rao DR. Alabama A&M University, Normal. PMID: 2099363

Pediatr Gastroenterol Nutr 1990 Nov; 11 (4):509-12. Effect of feeding yogurt versus milk in children with persistent diarrhea. Boudraa G, Touhami M, Pochart P, Soltana R, Mary JY, Desjeux JF. Service de Pediatrie, C. Oran, Algerie. PMID: 2262840

Nutr Cancer 1990; 14 (2):103-9 Effect of miso (Japanese soybean paste) and NaCl on DMBA-induces rat mammary tumors. Baggott JE, Ha T, Vaughn WH, Juliana MM, Hardin JM, Grubbs CJ. Department of Nutrition Sciences, University of Alabama, Birmingham. PMID: 2120681

Nourishing Traditions, Fallon S, Enig M. New Trends Publishing, 1999.

Cancer Res 1989 Ju15; 49 (14):4020-3. Consumption of fermented milk products and breast cancer: a case-control study in The Netherlands. van't Veer P, Dekker JM, Lamers JW, Kok FJ, Schouten EG, Brants HA, Sturmans F, Hermus RJ. Epidemiology Section, TNO-CIVO, Toxicology and Nutrition Institute, Zeist, The Netherlands. PMID: 2736542

Indian J Exp Biol 1989 Jan; 27 (1):72-5. Cytotoxic activity of lactobacilli isolated from plant and dairy sources. Manjunath N, Ranganathan B. PMID: 2606525

Chinese J of Prev 1989; 23 (6):352-4. A study on the effect of fermented soybean in prevention iron deficiency anemia in children. Qin HS. PMID: 2627849

Biochim Biophys Acta 1988 Dec 22; 946 (2):227-34. Lipid topology and physical properties of the outer mitochondrial membrane of the yeast, Saccharomyces cerevisiae. Sperka-Gottlieb CD, Hermetter A, Paltauf F, Daum G. Institut für Biochemie and Lebensmittelchemie, Technische Universität, Graz, Austria. PMID: 3061466

Immunology 1988 Jan; 63 (1):17-23. Systemic augmentation of the immune response in mice by feeding fermented milks with Lactobacillus casei and Lactobacillus acidophilus. Perdigon G, de Macias ME, Alvarez S, Oliver G, de Ruiz Holgado AP. PMID:3123370

J Dairy Sci 1986 Sep; 69 (9):2237-42. Antimutagenic properties of lactic acid-cultured milk on chemical and fecal mutagens. Hosono A, Kashina T, Kada T. PMID: 3097092

J Dairy Sci 1982 Dec; 65 (12):2388-90. Ion exchange separation of the antitumor component(s) of yogurt dialyzate. Ayebo AD, Shahani KM, Dam R, Friend BA. PMID: 7161436

Acta Micro Polonica 1977; 26 (3):281-4. Casein degradation and amino acid liberation in milk by two highly proteolytic strains of lactic acid bacteria. Chebbi NB, Chander H, Ranganathan B. PMID: 70973

Chapter Four
USP, Isolates, Mixtures and Probiotic Nutrients:
A Glossary of Commonly Misunderstood and Misapplied Terms

Curr Microbiol 2001 Ap;42(4):252-6. Microbiological and biochemical study of coffee fermentation. Avallone S, Guyot B, Brillouet JM, Olguin E, Guiraud JP. USTL F-34095, GBSA-MBI CC 23 Université de Montpellier II, Place Eugene Bataillon, 34095 Montpellier Cedex 5, France. PMID: 11178725

Science News 2001 Apr 21, 159 (16):248. High-selenium wheat protects against colon cancer in rats. (Abstract 78.7) Finley JW, Davis CD, and Hintze KJ, Experimental Biology 2001 Meeting. March 31-April 4. Orlando.

Cancer Epidemiol Biomarkers Prev 2001 Apr; 10 (4):385-390. Interactions of selenium compounds with other antioxidants in DNA damage and apoptosis in human normal keratinocytes. Shen CL, Song W, Pence BC. Texas Tech University Health Sciences Center, Lubbock, Texas. PMID: 11319180

Urology 2001 Apr; 57 (4 Suppl):185-187. Randomized, controlled chemoprevention trials in populations at very high risk for prostate cancer: Elevated prostate-specific antigen and high-grade prostatic intraepithelial neoplasia. Clark LC, Marshall JR. Arizona Cancer Center and Arizona College of Public Health, Tucson, Arizona. PMID:11295623

Enzyme Microb Technol 2000 Jul 1;27(1-2):127-133. Biological detoxification of coffee husk by filamentous fungi using a solid state fermentation system. Brand D, Pandey A, Roussos S, Soccol CR. Laboratorio de Processos Biotecnologicos, Departmento Engenharia Quimica, Universidade Federal do Parana (UFPR), 81531-970, Curitiba-PR, Brazil. PMID:10862912

J Nutr Sci Vitaminol (Tokyo) 1999 Jan; 45 (1):119-128. An evaluation of the bioavailability of selenium in high-selenium yeast. Yoshida M, Fukunaga K, Yasumoto K. Department of Biotechnology, Faculty of Engineering, Kansai University, Osaka, Japan. PMID: 10360246

JAMA 1996 Dec 25; (276) 24:1957-63. Effects of selenium supplementation for can-cer prevention in patients with carcinoma of the skin. A randomized controlled trial. Nutritional Prevention of Cancer Study Group. Clark LC et al. PMID: 8971064

Material Safety Data Sheet. MSDS Number S4946 2000 Apr. Sodium Selenite, 5-Hydrate. Mallinckrodt Baker, Inc. Phillipsburg, New Jersey.

Can J Microbiol 2001 Oct;47(10):935-42 Binding activity of natto (a fermented food) and Bacillus natto isolates to mutagenic-carcinogenic heterocyclic amines. Rajendran R, Ohta Y. Rajendran R, Ohta Y. Laboratory for Microbial Biochemistry, Faculty of Applied Biological Sciences, Hiroshima University, Highashi-Hiroshima, Japan. PMID: 11718547

Chapter Five
The Life Bridge
Section A – SELENIUM

J Urology 2001;166:2034-2038 Supplemental selenium may reduce prostate cancer risk. Westport, Connecticut.

National Institute of Health 2001 Aug. Dietary supplement fact sheets: Selenium. Clinical Nutrition Service, Warren Grant Magnuson Clinical Center, Office of Dietary Supplements, National Institute of Health.

Fresenius J Anal Chem 2001 Jun; 370 (2-3):286-90. Selenomethionine content of candidate reference materials. Wolf WR, Zainal H, Yager B. Food Composition Laboratory, BHNRC, ARS, USDA, Beltsville, Maryland. wolf@bhnrc.usda.gov PMID: 11451253

J Anim Sci 2001 Apr; 79 (4):942-8. Comparative effects of high dietary levels of organic and inorganic selenium on selenium toxicity of growing-finishing pigs. KimYY, Mahan DC. Department of Animal Sciences, The Ohio State University and The Ohio Agricultural Research and Development Center, Columbus, Ohio. PMID: 11325201

Urology 2001 Apr; 57 (4 Suppl):185-187. Randomized, controlled chemoprevention trials in populations at very high risk for prostate cancer: Elevated prostate-specific antigen and high-grade prostatic intraepithelial neoplasia. Clark LC, Marshall JR. Arizona Cancer Center and Arizona College of Public Health, Tucson, Arizona. PMID: 11295623

Science News 2001 Apr; 159:248. Anticancer mineral works best in food. Finley JW. Human Introduction, Food and Agriculture Organization of the United Nations, Rome 1999 Fermented Cereals A Global Perspective. Haard N, Odunfa SA, Lee C, Quintero-Ramirez R, Lorence-Quiñones A, Wacher-Radarte C. ISBN 92-5-104296-9

Biol Trace Elem Res 2000 Dec; 77 (3):273-85. Bioavailability and possible benefits of wheat intake naturally enriched with selenium and its products. Djujic IS, Jozanov-Stankov ON, Milovac M, Jankovic V, Djermanovic V. Institute of Chemistry, Technology and Metallurgy, Department of Chemistry, Belgrade, Yugoslavia. PMID: 11204469

J Nutr 2000 Sep; 130 (9):2384-9. Selenium from high selenium broccolli protects rats from colon cancer. Finley JW, Davis CD, Feng Y. US Department of Agriculture, Agricultural Research Service, Grand Forks Human Nutrition Research Center, Grand Forks, North Dakota, USA. PMID: 1095884

J Trace Elem Med Biol 2000 Jun; 14 (2):84-7. Effect of supplementation with organic selenium on mercury status as measured by mercury in pubic hair. Seppanen K, Kantola M, Laatikainen R, Nyyssonen K, Valkonen VP, Kaarlopp V, Salonen JT. Department of Chemistry, University of Kuopio, Finland. PMID: 10941718

J Agric Food Chem 2000 June; 48 (6):2062-70. Erratum in: *J Agric Food Chem* 2000 Sep;48(9):4452. Chemical Speciation influences comparative activity of selenium-enriched garlic and yeast in mammary cancer prevention. Ip C, Birringer M, Block E, Kotrebai M, Tyson JF, Uden PC, Lisk DJ. Department of Experimental Pathology, Roswell Park Cancer Institute, Buffalo, New York. Clement.Ip@roswellpark.org PMID: 10888499

J Trace Elem Med Biol 2000 Apr; 14 (1):43-7. Preparation of selenium yeasts I. Preparation of selenium-enriched Saccharomyces cerevisiae. Suhajda A, Hegoczki J, Janzso B, Pais I, Vereczkey G. Department of Agricultural Chemical Technology, Technical University of Budapest, Hungary. PMID: 10836533

J Anim Sci 1999 Dec; 77 (12):3371-6. The influence of dietary selenium as selenium yeast or sodium selenite on the concentration of selenium in the milk of Suckler cows and on the selenium status of their calves. Pehrson B, Ortman K, Madjid N, Trafikowska U. Swedish University of Agricultural Sciences, Faculty of Veterinary Medicine, Department of Animal Environment and Health, Skara, Sweden. Bo.Pehrson@hmh.slu.se PMID: 10641886

J Agric Food Chem 1999 Jun; 47 (6):2491-5. Production of organically bound selenium yeast by continuous fermentation. Demirci A, Pometto AL III. Department of Food Science and Human Nutrition, Iowa State University, Ames, Iowa. PMID: 10794655

J Nutr Sci Vitaminol (Tokyo) 1999 Jan; 45 (1):119-128. An evaluation of the bioavailability of selenium in high-selenium yeast. Yoshida M, Fukunaga K, Yasumoto K. Department of Biotechnology, Faculty of Engineering, Kansai University, Osaka, Japan. PMID: 10360246

Acta Vet Scan 1999; 40 (1):23-34. The influence of supplements of selenite, selante and selenium yeast on the selenium status of dairy heifers. Ortman K, Anderson R, Holst H. Department of Animal Environment and Health, Faculty of Veterinary Medicine, Swedish University of Agricultural Sciences, Uppsala, Sweden. K.Ortman@hmh.slu.se PMID: 10418193

Food and Agriculture Organization of the United Nations Rome 1999 Fermented Cereals A Global Perspective. Haard N, Odunfa S.A., Lee C, Quintero-Ramirez R, Lorence-Quiñones A, wacher-Radarte C. ISBN 92-5-104296-9

Biol Trace Elem Res 1998 Nov; 65 (2):143-51. Bioavailability of enteral yeast-selenium in preterm infants. Bogye G, Alffhan G, Machay T. National Institute of Rheumatology and Physiotherapy, Budapest, Hungary. PMID: 9881518

Med Klin 1997 Sep 15; 92 Suppl 3:42-5. Reduction of cancer mortality and incidence by selenium supplementation. Combs GF Jr., Clark LC, Turnbull BW. Division of Nutritional Sciences, Cornell University, Ithaca, New York. gfc2@cornell.edu PMID: 9342915

Biomed Environ Sci 1997 Sep; 10 (2-3):227-34. Reduction of cancer risk with an oral supplement of selenium. Combs GF Jr., Clark LC, Turnbull BW. Division of Nutritional Sciences, Cornell University, Ithaca, New York. PMID: 9315315

Reuters Health 1997 Feb 24. Effects of selenium for cancer. Clark L. Arizona Cancer Center, Tucson.

JAMA 1996 Dec; (276) 24:1957-63. Effects of selenium supplementation for cancer prevention in patients with carcinoma of the skin. Clark LC et al. PMID: .

Biol Trace Elem Res 1990 Jun; 25 (3):201-9. Study of the oxidative metabolic function and chemotaxis of neutrophils from patients with cancer influenced by selenium yeast. Xu HB, Mei WD, Dong ZM, Liao BL. Huazhong University of Science and Technology, Wuhan, People's Republic of China. PMID: 1698418

Annals of Medicine 1990 Feb; 22 (1):37-41. Lactic acid bacteria and human health. Gorbach SL. Department of Community Health, Tufts University School of Medicine, Boston, MA

Biol Trace Elem Res 1988 Jan-April; 15:125-38. Comparison of whole blood selenium values and erythrocyte glutathione peroxidase activities of normal individuals on supplementation with selenate, selenite, L-selenomethionine, and high selenium yeast. Clausen J, Nielsen SA. Institute for Life Science and Chemistry, University of Roskilde, Denmark. PMID: 2484510

Ann Clin Res 1986; 18 (1)65-8. Erratum in: *Ann Clin Res* 1986;18(4): Following 216: Selenium yeast. Korhola M, Vainio A, Edelmann K. PMID: 3521441

Section B – IRON AND COPPER

J Biol Chem 1999 July; 274 (27):18989-96. Mechanism of Iron Transport to the Site of Heme Synthesis inside Yeast Mitochondria. Lange H, Kispal G, Lill R. From the Institut fur Zytobiologie und Zytopathologie der Philipps-Universitat Margurg, Robert-Koch-Strasse 5, 35033 Marburg, Germany and the Institue of Biochemistry, University Medical School of Pecs, Szigeti 12, 7624 Pecs, Hungary. PMID: 10383398

Clinical Microbiology Reviews 1999 July; 12 (3)0893-8512. Acquisition, Transport, and Storage of Iron by Pathogenic. Howard D. Department of Microbiology and Immunology, UCLA School of Medicine, Los Angeles, California. PMID: 10398672

Nutr Rev 1999 Apr; 57 (4):114-123. Iron transport across biologic membranes. Andrews NC, Fleming MD, Gunshin H. Howard Hughes Medical Institute, Children's Hospital, Boston, MA. PMID: 10228348

Metal Ions in fungi 1994; 11:149-178. Reductive iron assimilation in Saccharomyces cerevisiae. Winkelmann G, Winge DR. Marcel Dekker, Inc., New York, NY.

FEBS Lett 1999 June; 452 (1-2):57-60. Mitochondrial assembly in yeast. Grivell LA, Artal-Sanz M, Hakkaart G, de Jong L, Nijtmans LG, van Oosterum K, Siep M, van der Spek H. Section for Molecular Biology, Institute of Molecular Cell Biology, University of Amsterdam, The Netherlands. PMID: 10376678

Section C – CHROMIUM

J Biosci 2001 Jun; 26 (2):217-23. Chromium uptake by Saccharomyces cerevisiae and isolation of glucose tolerance factor from yeast biomass. Zetic VG, Stehlik-Thomas V, Grba S, Lutilsky L, Kozlek D. Laboratory of Fermentation and Yeast Technology, Faculty of Food Technology and Biotechnology, University of Zagreb, Pierottijeva 6, 1000 Zagreb, Croatia. PMID: 11426057

J Agric Food Chem 2000 Feb; 48 (2):531-6. Enhanced organically bound chromium yeast production. Demirci A, Pometto III AL. Department of Food Science and Human Nutrition, 2312 Food Sciences Building, Iowa State University, Ames, Iowa. PMID: 10691671

Nippon Rinsho 1996 Jan; 54 (1):79-84. Role of essential trace elements in the disturbance of carbohydrate metaboism. Kimura K. Department of Biochemistry, Faculty of Medicine, Tottori University. PMID: 8587210
Biol Trace Elem Res 1992 Jan; 32:25-38. The isolation of glucose tolerance factors from brewer's yeast and their relation to chromium. Simonoff M, Shapcott D, Alameddine S, Sutter-Dub MT, Simonoff G. Recherche Fondamentale et Clinique sur les Elements-traces, URA 451 du CNRS, Gradignan, France. PMID: 1375061

J Inorg Biochem 1983 June; 18 (3):195-211 Seperation of Biologically active chromium-containing complexes from yeast extracts and other sources of glucose tolerance factor (GTF) activity. Haylock SJ, Buckley PD, Blackwell LF. PMID: 6409995

Section D – CO-ENZYME Q10
Vitam Horm 2001; 61:173-218. Biosynthesis of menaquinone (vitamin K2) and ubiquinone (coenzyme Q): a perspective on enzymatic mechanisma. Meganathan R. Department of Biological Sciences, Northern Illinois University, DeKalb, Illinois.

Analysis Report for Quercetin and COQ10 Products 2001 Apr. Vinson J.

Section E – VITAMIN C
Vitam Horm 2001; 61:241-66. L-ascorbic acid biosynthesis. Smirnoff N. School of Biological Sciences, University of Exeter, Exeter EX4 4PS, United Kingdom. PMID: 11153268

Vitam Horm 2001; 61:157-71. The biosynthesis of coenzyme A in bacteria. Begley TP, Kinsland C, Strauss E. Department of Chemistry and Chemical Biology, Cornell University, Ithaca, New York. PMID: 11153265

Emergency Medicine 2000 Nov;18 (4):709-22. Pharmacologic Advances in Emergency Medicine. Nelson L, Perrone J. W.B. Sauders Company. Medical Toxicology Felloship, New York City Poison Control Center. nycpcc@hotmail.com. PMID: 11130934

FEMS Microbiol Lett 2000 May 15;186. Biosynthesis of L-ascorbic acid (vitamin C) by Saccharomyces cerevisiae. Hancock RD, Galpin JR, Viola R. Scottish Crop Research Institute, Division of Biochemistry and Cell Biology, Unit of Plant Biochemistry, Invergowrie, Dundee, UK. PMID: 10802179

ABC News 2000 Mar 15; Study: Vitamin C pill may harden the arteries.

USA Today 2000 Mar 3: Study: Vitamin C pills may clog arteries.

Applied and Enviromental Microbiology 1999 Oct; 65(10)4685-87. Bacterial Production of D-Erythroascorbic Acid and L-Ascorbic Acid through Functional Expression of Saccharomyces cerevisiae, D-Arabinono-1,4-Lactone Oxidase in Escherichia coli. Lee BH, Huh WK, Kim ST, Lee JS, Kang SO. Laboratory of Biophysics, Department of Microbiology, College of Natural Sciences, and Research Center for Molecular Microbiology, Seoul National University, Seoul 151-742 Republic of Korea. PMID: 10508108

Am J Clin Nutr 1999 Jun; 69 (6):1086-107 Toward a new recommended dietary allowance for vitamin C based on antioxidant and health effects in humans. Carr AC, Frei B. Linus Pauling Institute, Oregon State University, Corvallis 97331, USA. PMID: 10357726

Rev Latinoam Microbiol 1999 Apr-June; 41 (2):91-103. (Article in Spanish) Potassium transport in yeast. Lopez R, Pena A. Departamento de Genetica y Biologia Molecular, Instituto de Fisologia cellular, UNAM, Mexico, D.F. ruthl@ifisol.unam.mx. PMID: 10970213

JAMA 1999 Apr 21; 281 (15):1415-23 Criteria and recommendations for vitamin C intake.Levine M, Rumsey SC, Daruwala R, Park JB, Wang Y. Molecular and Clinical Nutrition Section, Digestive Diseases Branch, National Institute of Diabetes and Digestive and Kidney Diseases, National Institutes of Health, Bethesda, MD 20892, USA. PMID: 10217058

Nature 1998 Apr; 392(6676):559. Vitamin C has Both Pro-Oxidant And Antioxidant Effects In Vivo. Podmore ID, Griffiths HR, Herbert KE, Mistry N, Mistry P, Lunec J. PMID: 9560150

Proc Natl Acad Sci 1996 Apr;93:3704-9. Vitamin C pharmacokinetics in healthy volunteers: Evidence for a recommended dietary allowance. Levine M, Conry-Cantilena C, Wang Y, Welch R, Washko P, Dhariwal K, Park J, Lazarev A, Graumlich J, King J, Cantilena L. National Institute of Diabetes and Digestive and Kidney Diseases, National Institutes of Health, Bethesda, MD. PMID: 8623000

Mol Endocrinol 1993 Jul; 7 (7):833-9. Positive regulation of the vitamin D receptor by its cognate ligand in heterologous expression systems. Santiso-Mere D, Sone T, Hilliard GM 4th, Pike JW, McDonnell DP. Ligand Pharmaceuticals, Inc. Department of Molecular Biology, La Jolla, California. PMID: 8413308

Mol Neurobiol 1992 Spr; 6 (1):41-73. Vitamin neurotoxicity. Snodgrass SR. Department of Neurology, University of Southern California, School of Medicine, Los Angeles. PMID: 1463588

Eur J Biochem 1982 Oct; 127 (2):391-6. Biosynthesis of ascorbate in yeast. Purification of L-galactono-1,4-lactone oxidase with properties different from mammalian L-gulonolactone oxidase. Bleeg HS, Christensen F. PMID: 6754380

Section F – CALCIUM

Discover 2000 Aug; 45-51. Worrying about milk. Hively W.

International Journal of Food Sciences and Nutrition 1999; 50.351-356. Calcium bioavailability of selected Egyptian foods with emphasis on the impact of fermentation and germination. Ghanem KZ, Hussein L. Department of Nutrition, National Research Center, Giza-Dokki, Egypt. PMID: 10719566

Am J Epidemiol 1997 May 15; 145 (10):926-934. Calcium intake and fracture risk: results from the study of osteoporotic fractures. Cumming RG, Cummings SR, Nevitt MC, Scott J, Ensrud KE, Vogt TM, Fox K. Department of Public Health and Community Medicine, University of Sydney, Austrailia. PMID: 9149664

Ann Intern Med 1997 Apr 1; 126 (7):497-504. Comparison of dietary calcium with supplemental calcium and other nutrients as factors affecting the risk for kidney stones in women. Curhan GC, Willett WC, Speizer FE, Spiegelman D, Stampfer MJ. Department of Nutrition, Harvard School of Public Health, Boston, MA. PMID: 9092314

Calcif Tissue Int 1992 Mar; 50 (3):261-5. Liposome interactions with hydroxyapatite crystals: a possible mechanism in the calcification of atherosclerotic plaques. Hirsch D, Landis Wj, Azoury R, Sarig S. Casali Institute of Applied Chemistry, Graduate School of Applied Science and Technology, Hebrew University of Jerusalem, Israel. PMID: 1617501

J Bone Miner Res 1989 Aug; 4 (4):469-475. Calcium absorption in women: relationships to calcium intake, estrogen status, and age. Heaney RP, Recker RR, Stegman MR, Moy AJ. Hard Tissue Research Center, Creighton University School of Medicine, Omaha, NE. PMID: 2816496

Clinical Pharmacy 1987 Oct; 6 (10):770-7. Evaluation of prenatal vitamin-mineral supplements. Newman V, Lyon RB, Anderson PO. Department of Reproductive Medicine, University of CA, San Diego Medical Center. PMID: 3505840

Section G – VITAMIN B

Vitam Horm 2001; 61:157-71 The biosynthesis of coenzyme A in bacteria. Begley TP, Kinsland C, Strauss E. Department of Chemistry and Chemical Biology, Cornell University, Ithaca, New York, USA. PMID: 11153265

Schlafly Growler 2001 Feb; The Bavarian monks of St. Francis of Paula, who brewed a style of beer that came to be known as "flüssiges Brot", or liquid bread. The Saint Louis Brewery and Tap Room, Volume 7, Issue 2, Feb. 2001.

J Biol Chem 2001 Apr 6;276(14):10794-800 Saccharomyces cerevisiae is capable of de Novo pantothenic acid biosynthesis involving a novel pathway of bcta-alanine production from spermine. White WH, Gunyuzlu PL, Toyn JH. Department of Applied Biotechnology, DuPont Pharmaceuticals Company, Wilmington, Delaware 19880-0336, USA. PMID: 11154694

Biol Pharm Bull 2000 Jan; 23 (1):108-11 Biosynthesis of thiamin under anaerobic conditions in Saccharomyces cerevisiae. Tanaka K, Tazuya K, Yamada K, Kumaoka H. School of Pharmaceutical Sciences, Mukogawa Women's University, Nishinomiya, Hyogo, Japan. PMID: 10706422

Ukr Biokhim Zh 2000 May-Jun; 72 (3):25-30 [Riboflavin biosynthesis in yeast as a model for estimating mechanisms of regulating synthesis of biologically active substances]. [Article in Ukrainian] Fedorovych DV. Borets'kyi Ir, Division of Regulatory Cell System of O. V. Palladin Institution of Biochemistry, National Academy of Science of Ukraine, viv. fedorovych@biochem.lviv.ua PMID: 11200471

J Nutr 1999 Feb; 129 (2S Suppl):490S-493S. Cellular uptake of biotin: mechanisms and regulation. Said HM. Medical Research Service, VA Medical Center, Long Beach, CA 90822, USA. PMID: 100064315

Mol Microbiol 1999 Jun; 32 (6):1140-52 Genetic redundancy and gene fusion in the genome of the Baker's yeast Saccaromyces cerevisiae: functional characterization of a three-member gene family involved in the thiamine biosynthetic pathway, Orente B, Fairhead C, Dujon B. United de Genetique Moleculaire des Levures (URA 1300 CNRS,

Food and Agriculture Organization of the Untied Nations Rome 1999 Fermented Cercals A Global Perspective. Haard N, Odunfa S.A., Lee C, Quintero-Ramirez R, Lorence-Quiñones A, Wacher-Radarte C. ISBN 92-5-104296-9

Mol Microbiol 1999 Jun; 32 (6): 1140-52 Genetic redundancy and gene fusion in the genome of the Baker's yeast Saccharomyces cerevisiae: functional characterization of a 3-mamber gene family involved in the thiamine biosynthesis pathway. Llorente B, Fairhead FC, Dujon B. Unite de Genetique Moleculaire des Levures (URA 1300 CNRS,*UFR927* Univ P. and M. Curie), Departement des Biotechnologies, Insitut Pasteur, 25 rue du Dr Roux, F-75724 Paris CEDEX 15, France. PMID: 10383756

J Chromatogr A 1998 Sep 25;822(1):59-66 Chromatographic determination of flavin derivatives in baker's yeast. Gliszczynska A, Koziolowa A. PMID: 9810711

Biochim Biophys Acta 1998 Jun 29;1385 (2):201-19 Thiamin metabolism and thiamin diphosphate-dependent enzymes in the yeast Saccharomyces cerevisiae: genetic regulation. Hohmann M. Department of General and Marine Microbiology, Goteborg University, Medicinaregatan 9C, S-41390 Goteborg, Sweden. hohmann@gmm.gu.se PMID: 9655908

FEBS Lett 1998 May 29; 428 (3):245-9 Saccharomyces cerevisiae mitochondria can synthesise FMN and FAD from externally added riboflavin and export them to the extramitochondrial phase. Pallotta ML, Brizio C, Fratianni A, De Virgilio C, Barile M, Passarella S. Dipartimento di Scienze Animali, Vegetali e dell' Ambiente, Universita del Molise, Campobasso, Italy. PMID: 9654142

FEBS Lett 1998 Mar 13; 424 (3):127-30 The yeast gene YJR025c encodes a 3-hydroxyanthranilic acid dioxygenase and is involved in nicotinic acid biosynthesis. Kucharczyk R, Zagulski M, Rytka J, Herbert CJ. Institution of Biochemistry and Biophysics, Polish National Academy of Sciences, Warsaw. PMID: 9539135

Biochimie 1997 Dec; 79 (12):787-98 The coenzyme A-synthesizing protein complex and its proposed role in CoA biosynthesis in bakers' yeast. Bucovaz ET, Macleod RM, Morrison JC, Whybrew WD. Department of Biochemistry, University of Tennessee, Memphis 38163, USA. PMID: 9523022

J Mol Biol 1997 Oct 17; 273 (1):114-21 Dual role for the yeast THI4 gene in thiamine biosynthesis and DNA damage tolerance. Machado CR, Praekelt UM, de Oliveira RC, Barbosa AC, Byrne KL, Meacock PA, Menck CF. Depto. De Biologia, Universidade de Sao Paulo, Brazil. PMID: 9367751

Mol Microbiol 1997 Aug; 25 (3):541-6 Regulation of inositol monophosphatase in Saccharomyces cerevisiae. Murray M, Greenberg ML. Department of Biological Sciences, Wayne State University, Detroit, MI 48202, USA. PMID: 9302016

Biosci Biotechnol Biochem 1997 Jul; 61 (7):1221-4 Thiamine increases expression of yeast gene. Ichikawa K, Shiba Y, Yamazaki M, Serizawa N. Biomedical Research Laboratories, Sankyo Co., Ltd., Tokyo, Japan. PMID: 9255989

Eur J Cancer Prev 1997 Mar; 6 Suppl 1:S43-5. Intestinal flora and endogeneous vitamin synthesis. Hill MJ. European Cancer Prevention Organization, Lady Sobell Gastrointestinal Unit, Wexham Park Hospital, Slough, Berkshire, UK. PMID: 9167138

Gastroenterology 1996 Apr; 110 (4):991-8. Folate synthesized by bacteria in the human upper small intestine is assimilated by the host. Camilo E, Zimmerman J, Mason JB, Golner B, Russell R, Selhub J, Rosenberg IH. University Hospital de Santa Maria, Servico de Medicinia 2, Lisbon, Portugal. PMID: 8613033

Plant Mol Biol 1995 Nov; 29 (4):809-21 Evidence for the thiamine biosynthetic pathway in higher plant plastids and its developmental regulation. Belanger FC, Leustek

T, Chu B, Kriz AL. Plant Science Department, Rutgers University New Brunswick, NJ 08903, USA. PMID: 8541506

Biochim Biophys Acta 1995 May 11; 1244 (1):113-6 Origin of the nitrogen atom of pyridoxine in Saccharomyces cerevisiae. Tazuya K, Adachi Y, Masuda K, Yamada K, Kumaoka H. Faculty of Pharmaceutical Sciences, Mukogawa Women's University, Hyogo, Japan. PMID: 7766645

Ann Nutr Metab 1994; 38 (3):123-31 Effects of dietary proteins and yeast Saccharomyces cerevisiae on vitamin B6 status during growth. Masse PG, Weiser H. Ecole de nutrition et d'etudes familiales, Universite de Moncton, New Brunswich, Canada. PMID: 7979165

J Bacteriol 1993 Dec; 175 (23):7702-4 Biosynthesis of biotin from dethiobiotin by the biotin auxotroph Lactobacillus plantarum. Bowman WC, DeMoll E. Department of Microbiology and Immunology, University of Kentucky, Lexington, Kentucky 40536-0084, USA. PMID: 8244941

Biochem Mol Biol Int 1993 Aug; 30 (5):893-9 Pyridoxine is a precursor of the pyrimidine moiety of thiamin in Saccharomyces cerevisiae. Tazuya K, Yamada K, Kumaoka H. Faculty of Pharmaceutical Sciences, Mukogawa Women's University, Hyogo, Japan. PMID: 8220238

J Bacteriol 1990 Oct; 172 (10):6145-7 Regulation of thiamine biosynthesis in Saccharomyces cerevisiae. Kawasaki Y, Nosaka K, Kaneko Y, Nishimura H, Iwashima A. Department of Biochemistry, Kyoto Prefectural University of Medicine, Japan. PMID: 2170344

Experientia 1987 Aug 15; 43 (8):888-90 Occurrence of thiaminase II in Saccharomyces cerevisiae. Kimura Y, Iwashima A. PMID: 3305065

Experientia 1986 Jun 15; 42 (6):607-8 Thiamine-binding activity of Saccharomyces cerevisiae plasma membrane. Nishimura H, Nosaka K, Sempuku K, Iwashima A. PMID: 3522266

Mol Cell Biochem 1980 Mar 20;30(1):7-26 Coenzyme A-synthesizing protein complex of Saccharomyces cerevisiae. Bucovaz ET, Tarnowski SJ, Morrison WC, Macleod Rm, Morrison JC, Sobhy Cm, Rhoades JL, Fryer JE, Wakim JM, Whybrew WD. PMID: 6247641

Nature 1980 Feb;283(5749):781-2. Vitamin B12 synthesis by human small intestinal bacteria. Albert MJ, Mathan VI, Baker SJ. PMID: 7354869

Prep Biochem 1980;10(3):331-45 Alternate procedure for the preparation of the coenzyme A-synthesizing protein complex of Bakers' yeast. Tarnowski SJ, Whybrew WD, Morrison JC, Bucovaz ET. PMID: 6997858

Z Lebensm Unters Forsch 1977 May 26;164(1):15-6 [Effect of storage on the vitamin B6 activity of foods (author's transl)]. [Article in German] Kirchgessner M, Kosters WW. PMID: 577642

Appl Environ Microbiol 1977 Dec;34(6):773-6 Production of vitamin B-12 in tempeh, a fermented soybean food. Leim IT, Steinkraus KH, Cronk TC. PMID: 563702

J Bacteriol 1976 Dec;128(3):855-7 Regulation of thiamine transport in Saccharomyces cerevisiae. Iwashima A, Nose Y. PMID: 791939

INDEX

ABOUT THE AUTHORS

Richard L. Sarnat, M.D. is a physician and surgeon maintaining his practice in Chicago, Il. He is the founder of Alternative Medicine, Inc., a leading integrative medicine network contracted with Blue Cross and Blue Shield, HMO of Illinois. Dr. Sarnat is the author of *Physician Heal Thyself: What Every Practitioner Should Know About Alternative Medicine* (1995). He is a member of the American Medical Association and the American Academy of Opthalmology. He was graduated from Washington University in St. Louis (A.B., Phi Beta Kappa), Rush Medical College in Chicago (M.D.), and completed his ophthalmic residency at Northwestern University. He lives with his wife Loree in Wilmette, Illinois.

Paul Schulick is a nationally prominent herbal researcher and health educator. He founded New Chapter, Inc. of Brattleboro, VT and Luna Nueva Organic Farms of La Tigra, Costa Rica, companies dedicated to herbal and nutritional formulations. He received certification as a master herbalist from the renowned Dr. John Christopher, and is the author of the best-selling book *Ginger: Common Spice and Wonder Drug* (1996), now in its third edition. Together with Thomas Newmark he co-authored *Beyond Aspirin: Nature's Answer to Arthritis, Cancer & Alzheimer's Disease* (2000), recognized as the leading text on the complementary treatment and prevention of disabling COX-2 inflammation. He lives in Brattleboro, VT with his wife Barbi and their two children, Geremy and Rosalie, just down the road from Rudyard Kipling's home in the Black Mountains of Vermont.

Thomas M. Newmark is President of New Chapter, Inc., helping to chart that company's direction with his old college buddy Paul Schulick. In fact, all the authors met at their alma mater, Washington University, over thirty years ago, and have maintained their close friendship over the years. Tom, Paul, and Dr. Sarnat are also co-owners of Luna Nueva Organic Farms in Costa Rica, reflecting their lifelong devotions to organic gardening and farming. Tom co-authored *Beyond Aspirin* in 2000, and continues to explore the scientific bases of complementary approaches to health. He lives with his wife Terry and their five children in St. Louis, MO, and he and Terry share a studio in their home where he writes and she works her magic as a botanical illustrator.